# Cardiopulmonary Symptoms in
## Physical Therapy Practice

Meryl Cohen

Theresa Hoskins Michel

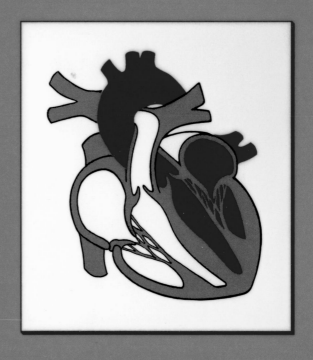

# Cardiopulmonary
# Symptoms in
## Physical Therapy Practice

## Meryl Cohen, M.S., P.T.

Adjunct Faculty, Program in Physical Therapy
MGH Institute of Health Professions at Massachusetts General
  Hospital
Certified Cardiopulmonary Specialist
Department of Physical Therapy, Cardiopulmonary Physical
  Therapy, and the Cardiovascular Health Center
Massachusetts General Hospital
Boston, Massachusetts

## Theresa Hoskins Michel, M.S., P.T.

Assistant Professor, Program in Physical Therapy
MGH Institute of Health Professions at Massachusetts General
  Hospital
Cardiopulmonary Clinician and Consultant
Department of Cardiopulmonary Physical Therapy
Massachusetts General Hospital
Boston, Massachusetts

**CHURCHILL LIVINGSTONE**
New York, Edinburgh, London, Melbourne  1988

**Library of Congress Cataloging in Publication Data**

Cardiopulmonary symptoms in physical therapy practice
    Meryl Cohen, Theresa Hoskins Michel.
        p.    cm.
    Includes bibliographies and index.
    ISBN 0-443-08558-7
    1. Heart—Diseases—Physical therapy.   2. Respiratory organs—
    Diseases—Physical therapy.   I. Cohen, Meryl.   II. Michel,
    Theresa.
        [DNLM: 1. Diagnosis, Differential.   2. Heart Diseases—diagnosis.
    3. Lung Diseases—diagnosis. 4. Physical Therapy—methods. WB 460
    C267]
    RC684.P57C37   1988
    616.1'2075—dc19
    DNLM/DLC                                                    88-18889
    for Library of Congress                                         CIP

© **Churchill Livingstone Inc.   1988**

Distributed in the United Kingdom by Churchill Livingstone, Robert Stevenson House, 1–3 Baxter's Place, Leith Walk, Edinburgh EH1 3AF, and by associated companies, branches, and representatives through the world.

Accurate indications, adverse reactions, and dosage schedules for drugs are provided in this book, but it is possible that they may change. The reader is urged to review the package information data of the manufacturers of the medications mentioned.

The Publishers have made every effort to trace the copyright holders for borrowed material. If they have inadvertently overlooked any, they will be pleased to make the necessary arrangements at the first opportunity.

Acquisitions Editor: *Kim Loretucci*
Copy Editor: *Kimberly Quinlan*
Production Designer: *Melanie Haber*
Production Supervisor: *Jocelyn Eckstein*

Printed in the United States of America

First published in 1988

# Preface

Physical therapy has expanded its role into a variety of new health care settings, including home health care, HMOs, and specialty practices. In all of these settings, therapists are seeing more complicated patients who have a constellation of medical diagnoses. The increased acuity of these patients and the recent exponential growth in medical technology place a burden on physical therapists to keep pace with current developments. Interpretation of new diagnostic procedures and management alternatives for patients with multiple diagnoses, including cardiopulmonary disease, have therefore become complex. Our book will assist the physical therapist in interpreting medical chart information and in deciding what, when, and how to evaluate cardiopulmonary symptoms in the patients they see.

This book contains three main sections. Section I provides an up-to-date review of cardiac and pulmonary symptoms—including anatomy, physiology, and pathophysiology—to aid the clinician in interpreting the database taken from a comprehensive chart review. These reviews will help the therapist in deciding what needs to be measured and in interpreting patient responses to physical therapy intervention. This section ends with a chapter on physical therapy evaluation techniques pertinent to patients exhibiting the symptoms described in subsequent chapters in this book.

Section II deals with nine symptoms. These major symptoms, all of which are frequently associated with cardiac or pulmonary problems, include chest pain, breathlessness, fatigue, irregular heart beat, loss of consciousness, cough, lightheadedness, edema, and leg pain. We have used a consistent format for presenting the information within each of these "symptom chapters," facilitating flow of information and cross-referencing between chapters.

Each symptom chapter begins with a table on the differential diagnosis of the symptom, followed by a chart review, which includes the medical history, physical examination data, and tests. The implications for physical therapy are presented throughout the discussion of the chart review. The medical–surgical interventions and indications for each symptom are then presented. Within this section, the discussion on rehabilitation deals primarily with the benefits of each component of a total rehabilitation program for the symptom being addressed. In the discussion on invasive monitoring

**v**

the commonly used evaluation or measurement techniques are described, and in invasive procedures the typical operations or special procedures used for symptom control or treatment are described.

Each symptom chapter ends with a general discussion on physical therapy intervention. In the discussion of the interview, key questions are provided for inclusion in the standard physical therapy interview. The evaluation focuses on musculoskeletal and cardiopulmonary procedures that are particularly relevant to the symptom. Functional evaluation and the way in which its findings may be used to design treatment programs are presented as well.

In the third section, typical case studies are examined, employing the strategies presented in this book. Each case study demonstrates a patient's "chronology of events" and encourages the use of clinical decision-making skills based on a clear understanding of patient diagnosis and clinical condition. Case data include pertinent history and intervention, patient responses to treatment, and interpretations of responses. The need for treatment modification is explained and subsequent outcomes are reassessed. The reader sees examples of how and what to measure, when measurements should be performed, and how to use the information obtained.

Our goal is to create a clinical reference to assist the physical therapist to confidently manage the patient with cardiopulmonary symptoms. A solid foundation gained from accurate interpretation of chart and patient information can better prepare the therapist to anticipate and prevent the provocation of these symptoms during physical therapy treatment. We hope that the ability to effectively treat more acutely ill and complicated patients who exhibit these cardiopulmonary symptoms will be enhanced by the use of this book.

*Meryl Cohen, M.S., P.T.*
*Terry Hoskins Michel, M.S., P.T.*

# Acknowledgments

Our gratitude goes to many unnamed colleagues who had encouraged us to pursue our goal of writing this book. Special thanks is extended to individuals who gave us their time and content expertise: Jill Downing, Harvey Simon, Ellen Anderson, Cynthia Zadai, Kate Grimes, and Marygrace Fiantaca. We are eternally grateful to our wonderful patients from whom we have learned invaluable lessons. Most of all, we wish to acknowledge the love and tireless devotion of our families and close friends, without which we would never have seen the fruition of this project.

# Contents

# OVERVIEW OF THE PULMONARY SYSTEM

# 1

## INTRODUCTION

Essential knowledge of the cardiopulmonary system will assist the physical therapist to distinguish between confusing symptoms that could arise from either pulmonary or cardiac dysfunction. Symptoms such as breathlessness, cough, or fatigue occur commonly. In order to appropriately treat these symptoms their etiology must be identified and understood.

## ANATOMY

Two components make up the pulmonary system: the gas-exchanging organ, i.e., the lungs and their constituent parts, and the musculoskeletal pump required to deliver the gas and remove it effectively.

### Gas-Exchanging Organ

The lungs may be visualized as an ''inverted tree'' made up of the airways beginning with the trunk; that is, the trachea divides at the level of the carina into the right and left main-stem bronchi, which subsequently divide into 25 generations, including the final air sacs, or alveoli, where gas exchange occurs. The vast surface area this network provides is said to be equivalent to a tennis court and suggests an immense reserve available for gas exchange. This inverted tree image, however, ignores the important structures of the nose, throat, and pharynx, which help to condition the air by filtering, warming, and humidifying it.

The lung tissue is made up of air sacs, capillary and bronchial networks, and a complicated blood vessel and bronchial branching system, with the branches coursing together from largest to smallest size. The resultant structure is an elastic, spongelike material, which normally is capable of a large degree of elastic recoil from a high degree of distensibility, or compliance. Within the thorax the lung is kept from collapse by a sealed membranous sac, the *pleura,* which maintains a negative pressure within the lung tissue so that it will not collapse. A puncture of the pleural lining will result in leakage of air into the cavity, which neutralizes the pressure against the atmosphere and results in a collapse called *pneumothorax.*

## The Musculoskeletal Pump

The term *musculoskeletal pump* refers to the thoracic cage and the muscles that contribute to the movement of air.

### Skeletal Components

The bony components of the musculoskeletal pump are the thoracic vertebrae, the ribs and their cartilaginous attachments, the sternum, the clavicles, and the scapulae. Misalignments of any of these parts will have an impact on the function of the musculoskeletal ventilatory pump. The ribs are set at specific angles relative to their vertebral connections (Fig. 1.1).

The particular shape of each rib and its angle of attachment help to determine the range of its movement with deep inspiration, and with forced full expiration. Normal rib motion includes three directions: up, out, and rotation. Some ribs shaped like the "bucket handle" rotate and swing outward. These motions provide space and suction for the internal passive lung tissue to move into.

### Muscular Components

The prime mover for inspiration is the diaphragm, which has its origin on the anterior and posterior aspects of the ribs, vertebral column, and ileum, and its insertion in the central tendon. It has a dual innervation, each side being separately innervated by the phrenic nerve, which controls the "hemidiaphragm." The contraction of this unique muscle generates a downward pull of the central tendon, thus pulling the inferior pleural sheath with it and creating the increased negative pressure within the cavity that draws air to the deepest portion of the lung as well as throughout all portions. External intercostal muscles contract simultaneously with the diaphragm to elevate and rotate the ribs with inspiration, allowing for air to move in anterior and posterior directions. In the absence of these muscles, as in quadriplegia, the stiffened ribs permit much less excursion and a reduction in the amount of air brought in for a maximal effort (vital capacity). The accessory muscles of breathing include the levator scapulae, the scalenes, the sternocleidomastoids, and the smaller throat muscles. These may be seen to be recruited

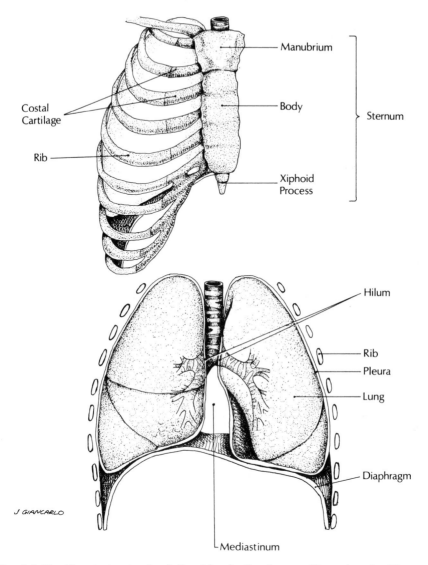

**Fig. 1.1** Significant structural relationships in the thorax. (Reproduced with permission from Shapiro BA: Clinical Applications of Respiratory Care. © 1977 by Yearbook Medical Publishers, Chicago.)

even in normal individuals during strenuous exercise. They become very significant muscles of inspiration when diaphragmatic function is impaired, as it is with chronic obstructive pulmonary disease (COPD). In the normal individual the thoracic muscles play a principal role in stabilizing the chest wall so as to optimize the conversion of diaphragmatic contractile tension to intrathoracic pressure and thus to volume change.[1,2]

## PHYSIOLOGY

### Gas Exchange

The pulmonary system functions in three primary ways: (1) It provides oxygen delivery from the atmosphere to the blood; (2) it provides for $CO_2$ elimination; (3) it protects the body from airborne invaders. In order to accomplish the gas exchanging functions both anatomic components must do their respective parts. The key to drawing a breath is creating an increasing negativity of pressure within the thorax (done by the muscles of inspiration), which creates the suction needed to bring atmospheric air into the airways. Getting it back out should be accomplished by a simple relaxation of all muscles, and the elastic recoil of the lung parenchyma will assist in release of the suction (or negative pressure) back to the original resting pressure, which is still less than atmospheric. Thus, expiration is a passive event during quiet breathing in the normal situation.

Once the air reaches the terminal airways, the membrane separating blood from gas is thin enough to allow for simple diffusion of $O_2$ and $CO_2$, which move in response to the concentration gradient. Since $CO_2$ is a much more easily diffusible gas than $O_2$, $O_2$ transport depends upon more factors than just the fraction in inspired air ($FiO_2$). The factors include the cardiac output, blood flow and distribution throughout the lungs and the periphery, hemoglobin concentration, and position of the oxygen dissociation curve. The last factor relates to the hemoglobin affinity for $O_2$, so that $O_2$ is more or less easily picked up or released to peripheral tissues. The curve is shown in Figure 1.2. It shifts to the right with an increase in temperature (fever) or decrease in pH (acidosis), which results in a decrease in hemoglobin affinity for $O_2$. A left shift occurs when the $PCO_2$ is low and the pH is high; it interferes with $O_2$ unloading to the tissues by increasing hemoglobin affinity.

### Mucociliary Escalator

One of the major functions of the lung is that of a body defense organ. It is capable of cleansing the body of invaders of all sorts, including dust particles, noxious gases, bacteria, and other microorganisms. It does not always succeed in ridding the body of infectious agents, and pneumonia is the result of a primary lung infection. However, the lung is equipped to combat a variety of offensive agents. Within the alveoli themselves there are phagocytic cells, which can engulf and digest certain invading organisms. Along the bronchial walls are special mucus-producing cells, which secrete mucus regularly. Mucus is a medium which collects particles. The cilia that line the bronchioles beat with a regular rhythm and clear mucus by sweeping it upward in the direction of the trachea. At the carina there is a sensitive

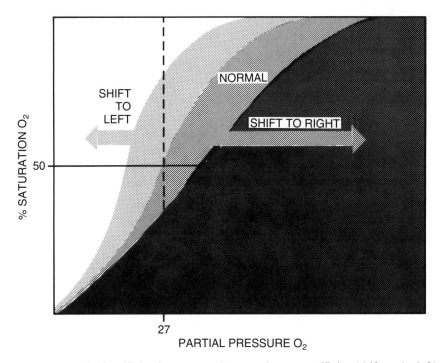

**Fig. 1.2** Hemoglobin affinity for oxygen. Increased oxygen affinity (shift to the left) means there will be a higher oxygen content at any given $PO_2$. Conversely, decreased oxygen affinity (shift to the right) means there will be a lower oxygen content at any given $PO_2$. (Reproduced with permission from Shapiro BA: Clinical Application of Blood Gases. © 1973 by Year Book Medical Publishers, Chicago.)

spot, which when stimulated produces cough. Cough obviously is designed to forcefully expel mucus and particles.

Effective coughing depends not only on an intact cough reflex itself but also on a strong, coordinated muscular response involving all the abdominal muscles, the internal intercostals, and even the back muscles in order to create a rigid chest wall, inside which can be built a high intrathoracic pressure that is used to expel substances.

## Muscles of Breathing

The diaphragm muscle has been extensively studied by pulmonary physiologists. Clearly, this muscle must demonstrate a high-endurance characteristic, since individuals must continue to breathe throughout their life spans yet must also demonstrate strength to be able to perform in response to exercise demands. The muscle fibers making up the diaphragm are primarily endurance type 1 fibers. The diaphragm will fatigue rapidly when a normal individual breathes against high resistance loads. The two primary factors that modify the strength of the ventilatory muscle contraction are the length-tension and force-velocity relationships.

### Length versus Tension

The familiar length-tension curve shows that the longer a muscle is before it contracts, the stronger the contraction that can be generated unless the muscle is overstretched. A shortened muscle cannot generate as effective a contractile force as an optimally lengthened one. Patients who have elevated residual volumes due to air trapping alter the starting length of the diaphragm in an unfavorable way such that the contraction will be weaker owing to a shortened length at rest of the diaphragm.

### Force versus Velocity

The force-velocity relationship indicates that the faster a muscle shortens, the less contractile force can be generated. At high respiratory rates, as with exercise, the speed of contraction may limit the strength of the diaphragm. Both strength and endurance of the muscles of ventilation have been shown to be trainable.[3]

## Work of Breathing

During quiet breathing of normal individuals at rest about 5 percent of the total body oxygen uptake goes to the muscles of ventilation and to the transport of gases and blood flow. For the same individuals doing maximal exercise, the demand for oxygen of the ventilatory system increases to no higher than 20 percent of the total. From these statements it is clear that normally the pulmonary function does not tax the body's ability to transport and utilize oxygen nearly as much as other bodily functions must. It is only in disease states that pulmonary function may become metabolically limiting to performance owing to escalation of the work of breathing. The components of the work of breathing are: (1) air flow resistance, (2) elastic tissue resistance, and (3) inertia of the system.

In exercise, when inspiration recruits more muscles of inspiration, including accessory muscles, there is an increase in the demand for oxygen. Furthermore, expiration, which at rest is a passive event, becomes active in maximal exercise, thus requiring additional oxygen consumption. As the respiratory rate increases, the force-velocity relationship requires that less contractile force be generated with higher speed of contraction. This causes less efficient muscle use. It also results in an increase in air flow resistance since with increasing rate of air flow, air moves with increasing turbulence and lessening laminar flow, especially in narrower or more tortuous airways. These normal adaptations with exercise account for the rise from 5 to 20 percent of the total oxygen uptake. In patients with restrictive or obstructive

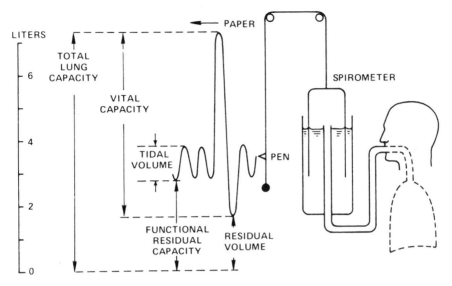

**Fig. 1.3** Pulmonary function testing. (Reproduced from West J: Respiratory Physiology. p. 13. Ventilation. Williams & Wilkins, Baltimore, 1979.)

lung disease, as will be discussed, a much higher percentage must be contributed to the work of breathing.

## Pulmonary Function Testing

The ability of the pulmonary system, i.e., the muscles of ventilation, to move air in and out of the thorax is measured with a spirometer. The subject simply breathes maximally in and out into a closed system, which permits a volume measurement over a calibrated time line (Fig. 1.3).

Volume measurements are made and used to determine the standard subdivisions of lung volume, which include total lung capacity (TLC), the vital capacity (VC), functional residual capacity (FRC), tidal volume (TV), residual volume (RV), inspiratory reserve volume (IRV), and expiratory reserve volume (ERV). The capacities are always made up of more than one volume (Fig. 1.4).

By means of forced breathing maneuvers, the air flow characteristics may also be assessed. The most informative test of air flow is a forced expiration, which simply shows how much air a patient can get out of his lungs as fast as he can push it out. The forced expiratory volume in 1 second ($FEV_1$) is a common measure of air flow, indicating how much air the patient moves out of his lungs in the first second of his forced expiration. Normal people can expel at least 80 percent of their total VC in the first second, but patients who have increased airway resistance, as those with obstructive lung disease, show a much lower delivery, often less than 40 percent of their VC in the first second (Fig. 1.5).

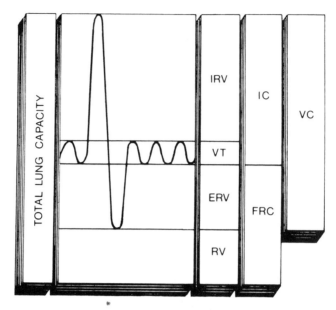

**Fig. 1.4** The divisions of total lung capacity. Total lung capacity (TLC) is the maximum amount of air the lungs can hold. The total lung capacity is divided into four primary volumes: inspiratory reserve volume (IRV); tidal volume (Vt); expiratory reserve volume (ERV); and residual volume (RV). Capacities are combinations of two or more lung volumes. They are inspiratory capacity (IC), functional residual capacity (FRC), and vital capacity (VC). (Reproduced with permission from Shapiro BA: Clinical Application of Blood Gases, © 1973 by Year Book Medical Publishers, Chicago.)

Patients who have restrictive lung diseases may deliver an unusually high percentage of the VC in 1 second and have much reduced VC as well. These variations from the norm make diagnostic evaluation from simple breathing maneuvers using a spirometer much more obvious. Values obtained from patients are always compared with predicted values derived from normative data based on subjects' age, sex, and body size. These factors clearly determine ventilatory muscle strength as well as thoracic cage dimensions. The range of variability is, however, quite wide, so that values within about 85 percent of those predicted are considered to be normal.

The maximal breathing capacity, often called the *maximal voluntary ventilation* (MVV), is a measure of strength of the muscles of ventilation. The patient must pant as fast and as deeply as he can for 15 seconds into a spirometer. The total volume of air he moves is his MVV. The major use of this parameter is in the maximal exercise test, when his maximal exercise minute ventilation or volume of air moved per minute (respiratory rate × tidal volume) is compared (as a ratio) with his MVV to see how much of his ventilatory reserve he needs to use to perform maximal exercise[3] (see Ch. 5).

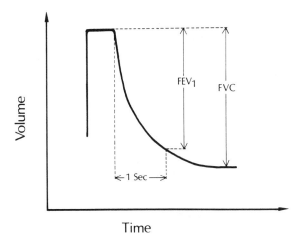

**Fig. 1.5** Schematic representation of a forced expiratory spirogram. Moving from left to right, a maximum inspiration is depicted by the rapid increase in volume (this represents inspiratory capacity). The patient holds his breath at maximum inspiration and then forces the air out as fast as possible. The total air expelled is the forced vital capacity (FVC); the volume expelled in the first second is the $FEV_1$. (Reproduced with permission from Shapiro BA: Clinical Applications of Respiratory Care. © 1977 by Yearbook Medical Publishers, Chicago.)

## Arterial Blood Gases

The amounts of oxygen and carbon dioxide in the blood determine the availability of oxygen to the tissues and therefore ensure healthy function of all body tissues. The partial pressure of oxygen in the blood ($PO_2$) is normally about 95 mmHg in young adults, with a range of 85–100, signifying normal hemoglobin and tissue perfusion. When the $PO_2$ drops below this range, there are four primary causes: (1) hypoventilation; (2) diffusion impairment in the lungs; (3) shunt (blood in the lungs does not pass by ventilated alveoli); and (4) ventilation-perfusion inequality. There may also be a fifth cause, which is the special case of high altitude or a lower than 21 percent $FIO_2$. With aging $PO_2$ may normally drop below that of younger people and may be as low as 60 mmHg without significant desaturation of hemoglobin.

The partial pressure of carbon dioxide in the blood ($PCO_2$) is an indication of the degree of metabolic activity in body tissues and is a primary determinant of blood pH.

## PATHOPHYSIOLOGY

There are two basic categories of pulmonary diseases with which we will be concerned, restrictive and obstructive lung disease. The term *restrictive lung disease* refers to conditions that limit the volume of the lungs, while *obstructive lung disease* comprises those conditions in which airflow characteristics are impaired. Some diseases, most notably emphysema, begin as obstructive but end with a restrictive component as well.

## Restrictive Lung Disease

Some restrictive lung diseases, such as sarcoidosis or pulmonary fibrosis, affect primarily the parenchyma, or lung tissue itself. In these cases normally compliant, springy, distensible lung tissue becomes thickened and fibrosed and loses elastic properties. The results are that the muscles of inspiration must work harder to distend lung tissue, there is less alveolar space available to support gas exchange, and the pulmonary reserve is limited. Consequently, patients may have sufficient lung surface area to support lower metabolic requirements for oxygen, as during low-level activities, but with exercise demands, the reserve is reached rapidly, and shortness of breath, with marked increase in respiratory rate, is found. This is due to the fact that the minute ventilation, which must increase during exercise, can only do so by an increase in respiratory rate if the TV is already at the maximum permitted by the amount of available lung tissue. On the pulmonary function test results, these patients show diminished volumes in all compartments of the lungs. However, air flow may be normal, or even higher than normal, since airways have normal integrity and usually function normally.

Another common form of restrictive lung disease involves alterations in the musculoskeletal pump. Neurologic conditions that limit the muscles of ventilation in their ability to develop contractile strength, such as the muscular dystrophies and quadriplegia, result in restrictive lung disease findings. In these cases lung tissue may be quite normal, but the ability to create sufficient negative pressures to fill all alveolar sacs is diminished. Lung function studies show reduction in lung volumes, including all compartments, since these tests depend upon volitional effort by the patient.

The other most common form of restrictive lung disease is that created by misalignment of the skeletal attachments that normally arrange the muscles of ventilation for optimal performance. Kyphoscoliosis is the most frequently encountered chest wall deformity that seriously diminishes lung volumes. However, any condition that may reduce rib cage mobility will ultimately reduce the amount of distention available to lung tissue. Severe obstructive lung disease does result in chest wall alterations, with stiff rib cages and barrel chest appearance as well as loss of alveolar space, so that lung volumes are also diminished through a restrictive component to the disease. The last form of restrictive lung disease worth mentioning is upper airway stenosis, such as ideopathic tracheal stenosis. In such cases less volume of gas is permitted past the stenotic section in the large airway, and measures of lung volumes show reductions consistent with restrictive lung disease.

# Obstructive Lung Disease

Obstructive lung diseases are commonly grouped together and referred to as COPD (chronic obstructive pulmonary disease). Included in this category are the specific disease entities of emphysema, chronic bronchitis, asthma, bronchiectasis, and cystic fibrosis.

## *Emphysema*

Patients with emphysema have abnormal enlargement of their alveoli due to the destruction of the gas-exchanging membrane, i.e., the walls of the alveoli. When the enlargement is so great as to be noticed on chest radiography, it may be referred to as *blebs* or *bullae*. This represents a loss of the elastic tissue of the lung, resulting in a less compliant lung structure. Patients may have a genetic disposition to emphysema owing to a deficiency of $\alpha_1$-antitrypsin, one of the lung protein enzymes. These are younger patients with very severe shortness of breath who may never have smoked cigarettes.

More typical is the emphysema patient who smoked cigarettes for many years, which did significant damage to several structures within the lung, including alveolar walls. One of the other structures that is permanently lost due to smoking is cilia lining the bronchial tree. Without cilia, the mucociliary blanket does not function, and secretions, particles, and infectious agents become lodged within the bronchial tree. Only gravity, manual techniques, and huffing and coughing may be successful in ridding the body of these substances before harm is done.

In part because of retained secretions, smaller bronchioles lose their wall integrity and become easily collapsible by external forces. When this happens, these small airways collapse during any forced expiratory maneuver, such as occurs with cough. In severe COPD premature airway collapse occurs, when expiration is no longer a passive, relaxed event but one driven by abdominal and intercostal muscle effort. Air is trapped in the large air sacs and blebs, which lack the elasticity to provide for a springback or elastic recoil of air during quiet expiration. It becomes a real problem to rid these lungs of old air. To do so, the emphysema patient begins to actively push air out of his lungs but, alas, often succeeds only in squeezing down on the bronchiolar walls because of the increase in intrathoracic pressure generated. Thus, air is trapped to an even greater extent. The act of expiration through pursed lips seems to provide for a back pressure within the bronchial tree, which prevents earlier airway collapse and the exacerbation of the air trapping problem. As more air is trapped within the thorax, there is a change in shape of the rib cage structure. Thus, the barrel chest appears, with the lower ribs flaring outwards and remaining distended. Since we recall that the diaphragm has its origin on these lower ribs, we realize that we have just flattened out the dome of the diaphragm by pulling it outward and downward. This is a permanent repositioning of the diaphragm, which places it at a mechanical disadvantage for achieving much contractile force as it strives to descend and bring in a full inspiration. With this new shortened length, reduced tension produces a loss of diaphragmatic strength, and some disuse atrophy of diaphragm muscle fibers may ensue. At autopsy patients with severe emphysema may show very little remaining muscle tissue, but rather a fibrous sheet where the diaphragm once attached.

As the diaphragm loses strength, it must also lose some endurance, yet the work of breathing for this patient has been increased by a number of mechanical changes, all of which lead to the sensation of breathlessness. These changes are:

More work of breathing because now expiration must be driven by muscular work.

Decreased efficiency of the diaphragm due to its flattened position and loss of full excursion so that it must require more energy to do less work.

Loss of elasticity by the lung tissue itself, which causes more work in distending the lung tissue in inspiration.

Greater air flow resistance within airways due to retained secretions.

A higher intrathoracic pressure required to move air in and out of the emphysematous lungs, with subsequent collapse of bronchiolar tubes.

With breathlessness, tendency of patients to breathe faster, approaching hyperventilation. At higher velocities of shortening, the muscular contractile forces are less, creating lower efficiency of contraction.

These factors all lead to an elevation in the work of breathing, for the COPD patients, which can become so severe that they are breathless even at rest and have no reserve for doing any exercise or functional activities at all. Activities that alter the position of the accessory muscles of breathing and end up supplementing the work of the diaphragm, such as placing arms over head, may be impossible for these severely affected patients. These tiny strap muscles are not efficient at performing the work of ventilating the lung and use a great deal of energy at this job compared with the diaphragm. However, by anchoring the shoulder girdle, these muscles are invoked during inspiration to provide for some assistance to the fatigued or flattened diaphragm. Patients always feel better when they lean forward on their arms to breathe.

### Chronic Bronchitis

Chronic bronchitis is clinically defined by the nature and frequency of the cough. Patients with chronic bronchitis almost always cough, but they may not realize it since it is second nature to them. The cough is stimulated by the presence of excess secretions in the bronchial tree. The mucus-secreting glands are hypertrophied, and there may be a larger number of these glands than found in the normal bronchial tree. This leads to the potential for airway obstruction, which occurs primarily in the conducting airways first but can lead to problems with the smaller airways and to emphysema. Since the most common etiology here also is cigarette smoking, emphysema and chronic bronchitis tend to coexist in many patients. Some patients have a dry, nonproductive cough but have severe emphysema. These people presumably have less of a chronic bronchitic component to their disease and tend to be very short of breath, but do not hypoventilate to the point that they show cyanosis or desaturation of their hemoglobin. Ultimately, if they lose all the available alveolar surface for gas exchange, they will desaturate, but this occurs with continued smoking or over a very long period of slow progression of emphysematous changes with aging. These patients are often referred to as "pink puffers." The patients who also have chronic bronchitis tend to retain $CO_2$ but owing to the kidney buffer system they maintain a normal pH with an elevation of $PCO_2$. These people may be less short of breath until exertion, but they do tend to desaturate, showing cyanosis. They also may be more likely to have right ventricular cardiac dysfunction due to the chronic elevation of vascular pressures in the pulmonary tree. For these reasons they are often called "blue bloaters."

## Asthma

Asthma is an airway disease caused by hypersensitivity of the smooth muscle within the bronchioles to external or internal stimuli. Smooth muscle will contract in response to an irritant factor, causing bronchospasm. Frequent episodes of bronchoconstriction may lead to hypertrophy of the smooth muscle and a constant stimulus to the mucus-secreting glands to supply more mucus. Asthmatic attacks may be very severe with hypersensitivity to a variety of factors or may be quite mild with rare sensitivity. During periods of remission, most pulmonary function test results are normal, but with illness the air flow tests show marked flow reductions. Typical stimulants for asthmatic sensitivity include allergens, infections, medications, exercise, emotion, and dust, animal hairs, or other environmental factors.

## Bronchiectasis

Bronchiectasis is characterized by dilatation of the bronchial tree. This is accompanied by excessive scretion of mucus, which often is thick and purulent and which often progresses to cellular infiltration and bronchial wall destruction. This leads to severe airway obstruction, with breathlessness on activity. Such patients have extreme susceptibility to infection.

## Cystic Fibrosis

Cystic fibrosis is a hereditary disease that affects the exocrine glands. In the lungs the mucous glands are affected and secrete thick, tenacious mucus constantly, which leads to their dilatation and fibrous atrophy. Bronchial plugs occur, which may occlude air flow and which certainly increase susceptibility to infection and inflammation. Mucociliary function is lost, and cough is the major mechanism of protection from lung infiltration. Eventual loss of alveolar surface area and similar chest wall changes occur with this disease, as was described for emphysema. Patients usually do not live beyond the age of 30, although with the advent of better antibiotic therapies some cystic fibrosis patients have been surviving into their forties. Musculoskeletal pump function failure with right ventricular cardiac failure is often the cause of their demise.[4]

## REFERENCES

1. Rochester D, Braun N: The Respiratory Muscles. Basics Respir Dis 6 (4):349 1978
2. Derenne J, Macklen P, Roussos C: The Respiratory Muscles: Mechanics, Control, and Pathophysiology. Am Rev Respir Dis 118:119, 1978
3. Leith D, Bradley M: Ventilatory Muscle Strength and Endurance Training. J Appl Physiol 41:1976
4. West JB: Respiratory Pathophysiology. p. 151. The Essentials. Williams & Wilkins, Baltimore, 1979

## SUGGESTED READINGS

Cash J (ed): Chest, Heart, and Vascular Disorders for Physiotherapists. Faber & Faber, London, 1975

Irwin S, Teckin J: Cardiopulmonary Physical Therapy. CV Mosby, St. Louis, 1985

Robbins S L, Cotran R, Kumar L, Pathologic Basis of Disease. 3d Ed. WB Saunders, Philadelphia, 1984

Shapiro B, Harrison R, Trout C: Clinical Applications of Respiratory Care. Yearbook Medical Publishers, Chicago, 1977

West J: Respiratory Physiology. Williams & Wilkins, Baltimore, 1979

# OVERVIEW OF THE CARDIAC SYSTEM

# 2

## ANATOMY

The heart is a four-chambered, muscular organ, which lies in the thoracic cavity. It is posterior to the distal two-thirds of the manubrium of the sternum, between the left and right lungs. Upon resection of the sternum the heart in its pericardial sac is visualized. On the surface of the heart muscle, imbedded in fatty tissue, are the coronary arteries. The right side of the heart lies most anteriorly. The chambers of the right and left sides of the heart are separated by an intramuscular septum, so that the left chambers are most posterior. The upper chambers, the atria, are connected to the lower chambers, the ventricles, by atrioventricular valves. These large, fibrous structures allow a unidirectional flow of blood from the atria into the ventricles. Cardiac anatomy is illustrated in Figure 2.1.

### Right Side of the Heart

Systemic blood enters the posterior aspect of the right atrium at two sites. The superior vena cava carries venous blood from the upper part of the body and is found on the upper right aspect of the atrium. The inferior vena cava brings venous blood from the lower part of the body and enters the heart at the inferior posterior border of the atrium. The coronary sinus, which carries deoxygenated blood out of the heart muscle, enters the atrium just anterior to the inferior vena cava. The right auricle, an extension of the anterior surface of the atrium and the endocardial surface of the anterior atrium, is lined with pectinate muscles, whereas the posterior portion of the atrium is smooth. The medial wall of the right atrium is formed by the muscular interatrial septum. An area of thinning and fibrous tissue, the fossa ovalis, lies in the septum and is a vestige of embryonic development.

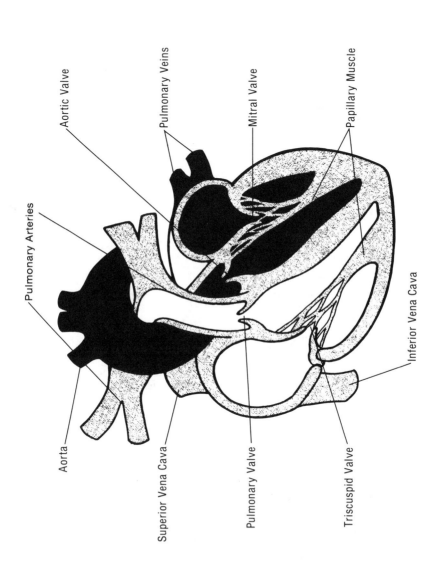

**Fig. 2.1** Inside of the heart. Note the position of the valves and their relation to the heart chambers and great vessels. Both atrioventricular valves are anchored to the ventricular wall by chordae tendinae and papillary muscles.

Aortic Valve

Pulmonary Veins

Mitral Valve

Papillary Muscle

Pulmonary Arteries

Aorta

Superior Vena Cava

Pulmonary Valve

Triscuspid Valve

Inferior Vena Cava

The base of the atrium is formed by the tricuspid valve, which is made up of anterior, posterior, and medial leaflets. This provides a path for blood to flow into the ventricle and is found posterolateral and to the right of the right ventricular outflow tract. The leaflets of the tricuspid valve are anchored to the muscular walls of the ventricle by the chordae tendineae of the papillary muscles.

The right ventricle is larger than the atrium, with thin muscle walls. Blood passes out of the right ventricle into the pulmonary artery trunk and into the lungs after crossing the pulmonary valve. This semilunar valve has three cusps (anterior, right, and left) and lies most anteriorly of the four valves in the heart. The pulmonary trunk lies next to the aorta in the left ventricle (Fig. 2.1).

## Left Side of the Heart

Oxygenated blood enters the left atrium via four pulmonary veins. The two veins from the right lung enter the left atrium just adjacent to the interatrial septum, and the two veins from the left lung enter the posterolateral aspect of the left atrium. The endocardial surface of the atrium is smooth except for the pectinate muscles of the left auricular appendage.

The base of the atrium is formed by the mitral valve, a large bicuspid valve made up of anterior and posterior cusps. This valve is anchored to the muscular walls of the left ventricle by the chordae tendineae of the respective anterior and posterior papillary muscles. The mitral valve, providing the unidirectional flow of blood into the ventricle, lies posterolaterally to the aortic outflow tract of the ventricle.

The muscular walls of the left ventricle, the major pumping chamber of the heart, are three times as thick as those of the right ventricle. Blood leaves the left ventricle through the aortic valve into the aorta and systemic circulation. The aortic valve, a semilunar valve like the pulmonary valve, has three cusps, the right, left, and posterior.

## Coronary Arteries

Oxygenated blood is supplied to the myocardium by the coronary arteries. The right and left coronary ostia are immediately distal to the right and left aortic valve cusps (coronary cusps) and give rise to the right and left coronary arteries.

The right coronary artery (RCA) travels in the fat pad along the right atrioventricular surface. There are two major branches at the right lateral border, the right marginal artery along the border of the right ventricle and the posterior descending artery (PDA), which travels around to the posterior aspect of the heart. When the RCA is dominant, the PDA is a major branch. It travels to the crux of the heart and then turns distally along the interventricular groove to the apex of the heart. The PDA provides blood supply to the posterior third of the interventricular septum, the atrioventricular

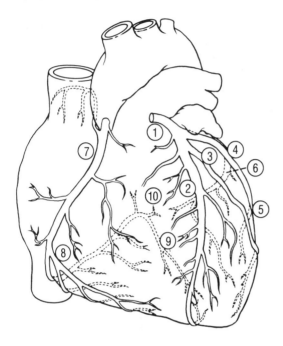

**Fig. 2.2** Coronary artery (CA) anatomy. (1) Left main CA; (2) left anterior descending CA; (3) diagonal branch of 2; (4) left circumflex CA; (5) marginal branch of 4; (6) posterior circumflex CA; (7) right CA; (8) marginal branch of 7; (9) posterior descending artery; (10) crux of the heart. (Adapted from Amsterdam E, Wilmore J, DeMaria A: Exercise in Cardiovascular Health and Disease. Reprinted from Yorke Medical Books, The Cahner's Publishing Company, a Division of Reed Publishing USA. New York, 1977.)

node, and a portion of the inferior-posterior fascicle of the left bundle branch (see description of conduction system below). Parallel branches of both the marginal artery and the PDA supply the walls of the right ventricle. Important branches of the RCA near its aortic orifice are the nodal and anterior atrial arteries. The former branch provides blood supply to the sinoatrial node, and the latter provides blood to the right atrium. In 60 to 70 percent of the population the RCA is the dominant coronary artery and provides the blood supply to the apex. In the remaining population either distal segments of the right and left coronary artery anastomose at the apex, or only a segment of the left coronary artery reaches the apex.[1]

The left main coronary artery (LMCA) quickly divides into two arteries. The left anterior descending artery (LAD) provides blood to the left ventricle, the anterior two-thirds of the interventricular septum, and conduction tissue, including the bundle of His, the right bundle branch, and the left anterior superior fascicle of the left bundle branch (see below under conduction system). The LAD also provides blood to the left anterior papillary muscle.

The second major branch of the LMCA is the left circumflex artery, which travels to the left lateral border along the atrioventricular groove to the posterior aspect of the heart. It sends arterial branches to the left atrium, the lateral wall of the left ventricle, a portion of the inferior posterior fascicle of the left bundle branch, and, occasionally, the left posterior papillary muscle.

Coronary artery anatomy is illustrated in Figure 2.2.

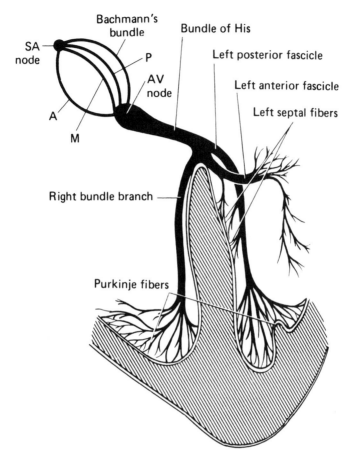

**Fig. 2.3** The conduction system. A, M, and P are the anterior, medial, and posterior interatrial tracts. (Reproduced from Goldman MJ: Principles of Clinical Electrocardiography. 10th Ed. © by Lange Medical Books, Los Altos, CA, 1979.)

## Conduction System

The heart has unique conduction tissue, capable of generating and rapidly transmitting electrical impulses, which cause its muscular walls to contract. The sinoatrial node (SA), or the "pacemaker" of the heart, is found at the junction of the superior vena cava and the right atrium. Three internodal pathways (anterior, posterior, and middle tracts) and Bachman's bundle travel through the atria to the base of the right atrium at the atrioventricular border and interventricular septum. The atrioventricular node (AV) continues distally for a short distance as the common bundle of His and then divides into the right and left bundle branches. These travel subendocardially along respective sides of the interventricular septum, with the left bundle branch

(LBB) dividing into two fascicles, the anterior superior and posterior inferior. These two fascicles and the right bundle branch (RBB) divide into Purkinje fibers, which are found throughout the myocardium. The continuous conduction system is illustrated in Figure 2.3.

## Cardiac Innervation

Both the sympathetic and parasympathetic nervous systems innervate the heart. Sympathetic nervous system (SNS) efferent fibers originate in the thoracolumbar region, travel through the superior, middle, and inferior cervical ganglia, and are received in the atria and ventricles. There are two types of sympathetic nervous system receptors, $\alpha$ and $\beta$, but only $\beta$ receptors, specifically $\beta_1$ receptors, are found in the heart. The catecholamines epinephrine, norepinephrine, and dopamine are the neurotransmitters for the SNS. The parasympathetic nervous system (PNS) efferent fibers traverse the vagus nerve and supply the atria and the SA and AV nodes. Acetylcholine is the primary neurotransmitter for the PNS. Both the PNS and SNS have afferent fibers that send impulses from the heart and great vessels to higher centers in the brain.

## PHYSIOLOGY

The function of the heart is to pump deoxygenated blood to the lungs and to pump oxygenated blood to all body tissues. It does this by a strong, synchronized ventricular contraction (systole). The characteristics of the contraction, including its frequency, strength, and volume ejected, are a result of the dynamic interaction of numerous physiologic principles. In normal man, continual, involuntary, and complementary regulatory systems work to ensure adequate tissue oxygenation for minimal through maximal metabolic requirements. Natural and/or pathologic factors can limit any part of the oxygen delivery system. The amount of oxygen required for metabolism is called the *oxygen consumption.*

Oxygen consumption ($\dot{V}O_2$) can be expressed by the following formula:

$$\dot{V}O_2 = \dot{Q} \times C\,(a - \bar{v})\,O_2$$

where $\dot{Q}$ is the cardiac output (i.e., the amount of blood that can be pumped through the body each minute) and $C\,(a - \bar{v})\,O_2$ is the arteriovenous oxygen difference (i.e. the amount of oxygen extracted by the tissues). Arterial oxygen minus venous oxygen content reflects oxygen that is taken up for tissue metabolism. An example of normal values at rest and during vigorous exercise follows:

$$\dot{Q} \qquad \times \; C \, (a \, - \, \bar{v})O_2 \; = \qquad \dot{V}O_2$$

Rest:     4,900 ml/min $\times$     40 ml/L   =   1.96 L/min

Exercise: 28,000 ml/min $\times$    120 ml/L   =   33.6 L/min

When stressed, the normal heart can increase its output to five to six times its resting capacity.

Cardiac output can be expressed by the following formula:

$$\dot{Q} \; = \; HR \, \times \, SV$$

where HR is the heart rate or frequency of contraction and SV is the stroke volume, which is the volume of blood ejected with each contraction. An example of normal values at rest or during vigorous exercise follows:

$$HR \qquad \times \qquad SV \qquad = \qquad \dot{Q}$$

Rest:   70 beats/min $\times$   70 ml/beat =   4,900 ml/min

Exercise: 200 beats/min $\times$ 140 ml/beat = 28,000 ml/min

The heart tissue has several basic properties that enable it to provide an effective output to meet body demands; these are automaticity, excitability, conductivity, and contractility.

## Automaticity

*Automaticity* is the property of the conduction tissue of the heart that enables it to spontaneously initiate an action potential. At rest, there is an electrical potential difference across cell membranes, causing them to be polarized. This is due to intracellular and extracellular potassium and sodium imbalance. The specialized conduction tissue of the heart allows sodium to slowly "leak" across its cellular membrane, eliminating this ionic imbalance, "depolarizing" the cell, and causing the action potential. At a certain threshold concentration the cell quickly becomes impermeable to sodium, again, reestablishing polarity across the membrane. The tissue of the SA node achieves the threshold for repolarization faster than any other part of the heart's conduction tissue, which is why this node is called the pacemaker of the heart. Secondary pacemakers along the conduction pathway of the heart can spontaneously initiate depolarization when the SA node fails, with

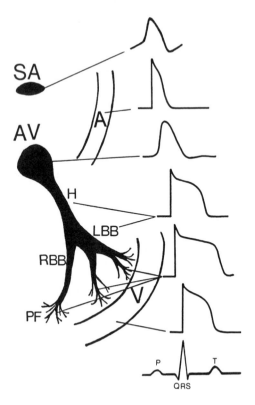

**Fig. 2.4** Diagrammatic picture of the conduction system of the heart. Cellular action potentials from various regions differ in duration, shape, and voltage range. SA, Sinoatrial node; A, atrium; AV, atrioventricular node; H, bundle of His; LBB, left bundle branch; RBB, right bundle branch; PF, Purkinje fibers; V, ventricle. The corresponding ECG tracing is shown at the bottom. (Reproduced from Thys D, Kaplan J (eds): The ECG in Anesthesia and Critical Care. Churchill Livingstone, New York, 1987.)

the more distal Purkinje fibers being the slowest to respond. Myocardial cells can spontaneously depolarize as well, but their action is even slower.

## Excitability

Excitability is the ability of cardiac tissue to respond to an impulse. An action potential in one cardiac cell can provide a stimulus to its neighboring cell and depolarize it. When the cell is not fully repolarized, it is unable to respond to a stimulus and is in its *refractory period*.

## Conductivity

Conductivity is the property of the heart that allows the impulse to spread throughout the specialized conduction system and myocardial cells. The velocity of impulse conduction varies within the heart, with the slowest conduction at the AV node and the fastest impulse conduction in the Purkinje fibers.

The electrocardiogram (ECG) is a graphic record of electrical impulses generated by the conduction tissue of the myocardium. It is a summation

| 1 | 23 | AVR-AVL-AVF | V1-V2-V3 | V4-V5-V6 |

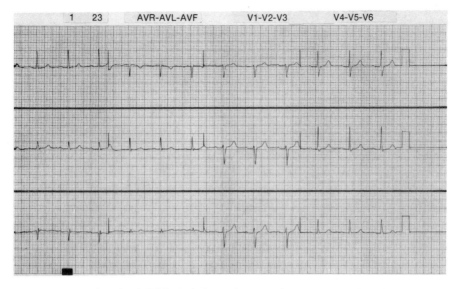

**Fig. 2.5** Normal 12-lead ECG. Labels at the top of each column identify the three leads displayed in the column.

of the waveforms produced from all heart tissue (Fig. 2.4). Negative and positive electrodes are placed on the skin on opposite sides of the heart to produce a typical complex of waveforms indicating atrial and ventricular depolarization and ventricular repolarization. The components of the waveform are the P, QRS, and T segments, labeled in Figure 2.4. The different but normal P, QRS, and T wave configurations in Figure 2.5 are obtained by altering the location of the negative and/or positive electrode on the skin to achieve 12 "views" of the heart. This allows more specific observation of the electrical activity of many parts of the heart muscle. The larger the positive wave deflection (above the isoelectric line), the greater the electrical activity in the direction of the positive electrode. Conversely, a negative wave deflection (below the isoelectric line) indicates that most of the myocardial cell depolarization is directed away from the positive electrode. Owing to the anatomic position of the left ventricle in the body, most electrical impulses in the frontal plane are directed down (caudally) and to the left (laterally) of the midline, accounting for the greatest positive deflections in lead II and negative deflections in lead aVR (Fig. 2.6). In the horizontal plane most myocardial electrical activity is directed anterolaterally, giving the greatest positive graphic deflections in V5 (Fig. 2.7).

The graphic representation provided by the ECG verifies the presence of the electrical properties of automaticity, excitability, and conductivity of heart tissue. It does not, however, reflect the heart's mechanical activity.

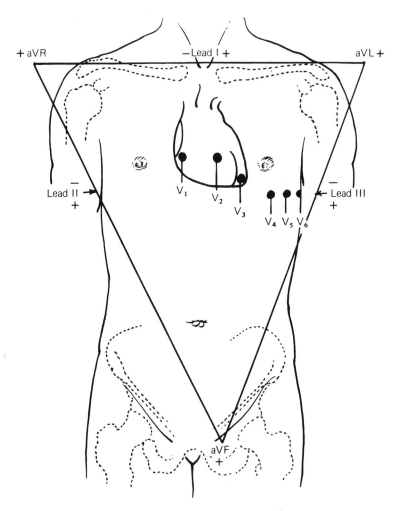

**Fig. 2.6** Graphic location of standard leads (I, II, III), unipolar limb leads (aVL, aVR, aVF), and unipolar precordial leads (V1–6) with reference to the heart. Polarity of surface electrodes of limb leads is indicated. The view of the wave of depolarization is seen from negative to positive electrode. (Reproduced from Krupp M, Sweet N, Jawetz E, et al. (eds): Physician's Handbook. 18th Ed. © by Lange Medical Books, Los Altos, CA 1976.)

## Contractility

Contractility is the property of heart muscle that enables muscle fibers to shorten. The myocardial cells, like skeletal muscle, contain actin and myosin myofilaments. The presence of calcium and adenosine triphosphate (ATP) in the cell allows the excitation-contraction coupling of these myofilaments

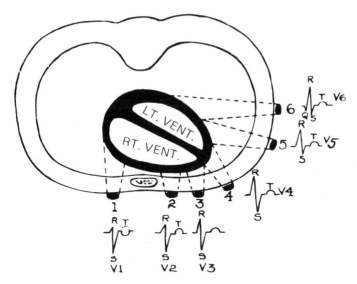

**Fig. 2.7** Precordial leads in relation to the chambers of the heart. (Reproduced from Krupp M, Sweet N, Jawetz E , et al (eds): Physician's Handbook. 18th Ed. © by Lange Medical Books, Los Altos, CA, 1976.)

to occur. Calcium enters the cell when the cell membrane is depolarized. Intracellular calcium is also required for cessation of this process and subsequent muscle relaxation.

The sequence of impulse generation and muscle contraction occurs spontaneously and repeatedly outside the body when the heart is bathed in a proper electrolyte solution. Within the body this sequence produces the clinical finding of a regular heart beat or pulse.

The atria depolarize slightly before the ventricles; therefore atrial contraction occurs slightly before ventricular contraction. Filling of the atria is primarily passive, while blood flow to the ventricles is a result of both passive filling and active contraction of the atria. The heart valves ensure that when heart chambers contract, blood flows in the proper direction. Once blood passes through a valve, the pressure generated by the volume of blood downstream from the valve forces the valve to close. When the heart is resting (diastole), the atrioventricular valves are open, allowing blood to fill the ventricles while the semilunar valves are closed. The pressure created by the blood volume in the ventricles causes the atrioventricular valves to shut and the semilunar valves to open as the muscle contracts and ejects its contents into the great vessels (systole). The flow of blood into the peripheral arteries correlates with palpation of peripheral pulses. One cardiac cycle is represented in Figure 2.8.

Note the relationship of electrical (ECG) hemodynamic (volume and pressure changes), and mechanical (heart sounds) events as time passes. A

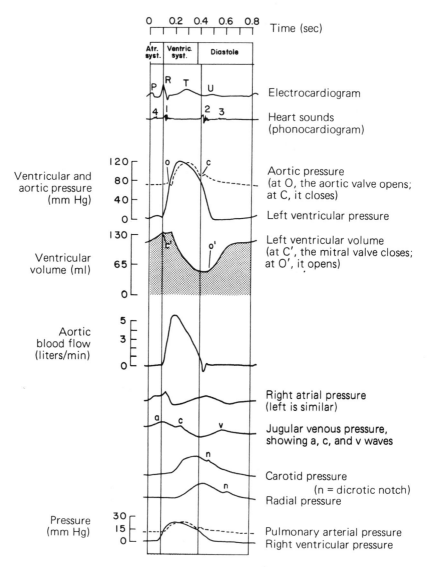

**Fig. 2.8** Events of the cardiac cycle. (Adapted from Ganong W: Review of Medical Physiology. 8th Ed. © by Lange Medical Books, Los Altos, CA, 1977.)

slight increase in ventricular pressure occurs after the P wave and a large increase in ventricular pressure occurs after the QRS complex. When ventricular pressure is great enough to open the semilunar valve, a large volume of blood leaves the ventricle and enters the aorta or pulmonary artery, as illustrated by the blood flow, volume, and pressure waves. When blood volume returns from the periphery or from the lungs, there is an increase

Table 2.1 Normal Cardiac Pressures

| Site | Systolic Pressure (mmHg) | Diastolic Pressure (mmHg) | Mean Pressure (mmHg) |
|---|---|---|---|
| Right atrium | 5–7 | 3 | <5 |
| Right ventricle | <25 | 3–7 | Not applicable |
| Pulmonary artery | <25 | <15 | <18 |
| Left atrium (direct or indirect wedge) | 10 | 7 | <10 |
| Left ventricle | 120 | 7–12 | Not applicable |
| Aorta | 120 | 80 | 90 |

in jugular venous pressure and then in atrial pressure. This pressure drops as the volume enters the ventricle. Normal pressures are listed in Table 2.1.[2]

The quality, or force, of the heart's contraction is influenced by many factors, including blood characteristics, autonomic nervous system, external influences such as exercise, and the presence or absence of pathology. Clinically, the strength of myocardial contraction is measured as the blood pressure (BP). The systolic blood pressure (SBP) is the force with which the heart propels blood into the periphery. The pressure required to maintain arterial patency while the heart rests is the diastolic blood pressure (DBP). Both are measured in millimeters of mercury.

## Determinants of Blood Pressure

Blood pressure can be considered as the product of the cardiac output ($\dot{Q}$) and total peripheral resistance (TPR).[3] A diagramatic representation of the factors that determine systemic arterial pressure can be found in Figure 2.9.

### Cardiac Output

As discussed earlier in this chapter, $\dot{Q} = HR \times SV$. At rest the heart rate, determined by the frequency of sinus node depolarization, is set by the balance of attempts by the SNS to accelerate and by the PNS to depress

Table 2.2 Cardiac Response to Autonomic Nervous System Stimulation

| Anatomy | Cholinergic Stimulation (PNS)[a] | Adrenergic Stimulation (SNS)[a] |
|---|---|---|
| Sinoatrial node | Decrease heart rate Vagal arrest | Increase heart rate |
| Atria | Decrease in contractility Increase in conduction velocity (usually) | Increase in contractility Increase in conduction velocity |
| Atrioventricular node and conduction system | Decrease in conduction velocity Atrioventricular block | Increase in conduction velocity |
| Ventricles | | Increase in contractility Increase in conduction velocity |

[a] PNS and SNS refer to the parasympathetic and sympathetic nervous systems, respectively.

(Adapted from Ganong W, Review of Medical Physiology, 8th Ed. © by Lange Medical Books, Los Altos, CA, 1977.)

the pacemaker's function. Table 2.2 lists the specific heart responses to adrenergic (SNS) and cholinergic (PNS) impulses.

The stroke volume (SV), which is defined as the difference between end diastolic volume (EDV) and end systolic volume (ESV), is dependent on several factors.

The EDV reflects the amount of blood entering the heart from the veins

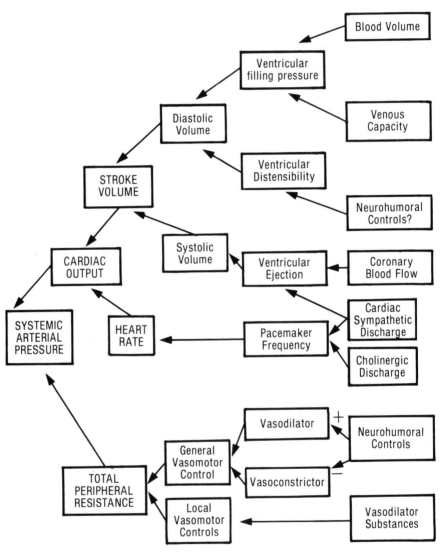

**Fig. 2.9** Factors determining systemic arterial pressure. (Modified from Rushmer R: Cardiovascular Dynamics. 4th Ed. WB Saunders, Philadelphia, 1976. Reprinted with permission from WB Saunders Co.)

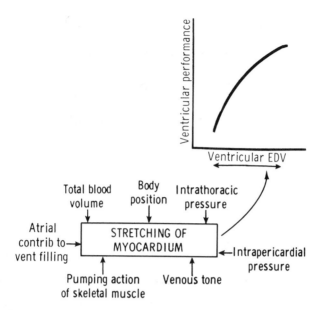

**Fig. 2.10** Relation between ventricular end diastolic volume (EDV) and ventricular performance (Frank-Starling curve), with a summary of the major factors affecting EDV. (Reproduced from Braunwald E, Ross J, Sonnenblick EH: Mechanisms of contraction of the normal and failing heart. N Engl J Med 277:794, 1967.)

(preload). Veins can distend and constrict. Distention allows for an improved ability to hold large volumes of blood, whereas constriction, occurring with smooth muscle contraction, allows for maintenance of tone. Preload depends on intravascular fluid volume and adequate distensibility of the chambers to accommodate the entering blood volume. The greater the volume entering the normal heart, the greater the stretch of the myocardium and consequently the larger the EDV. Figure 2.10 shows factors contributing to preload.

Cardiac muscle maintains similar properties to skeletal muscle in that as muscle is stretched, more tension is generated. The Frank-Starling law of the heart states that the "energy of contraction is proportional to the initial length of the cardiac muscle fiber." The curve in Figure 2.10 demonstrates this relationship.

In addition to the degree of stretch of the heart muscle, autonomic stimulation and coronary blood flow affect its contractility. As can be seen in Table 2.2, the force of myocardial contraction, or *inotropy,* is increased by SNS stimulation of both atria and ventricles while the PNS decreases atrial contractility. Coronary artery blood flow provides the myocardium with the oxygen it needs for metabolic processes and the energy to contract.

Stimulation of $\beta_2$ receptors in the coronary arteries produces vasodilation whereas stimulation of $\alpha$ receptors in the coronary arteries causes

**Table 2.3 Blood Vessel Responses to Autonomic Nervous System Stimulation**

| Blood vessel | Cholinergic Impulse Response | Adrenergic Impulse Response | |
|---|---|---|---|
| | | Receptor | Type |
| Coronary | Dilation | $\alpha$ | Constriction |
| | | $\beta_2$ | Dilation |
| Skin and mucosa | — | $\alpha$ | Constriction |
| Skeletal muscle | Dilation | $\alpha$ | Constriction |
| | | $\beta_2$ | Dilation |
| Cerebral | — | $\alpha$ | Constriction (slight) |
| Pulmonary | — | $\alpha$ | Constriction |
| Abdominal viscera | — | $\alpha$ | Constriction |
| | | $\beta_2$ | Dilation |
| Renal | — | $\alpha$ | Constriction |
| Salivary glands | Dilation | $\alpha$ | Constriction |

(Adapted from Ganong W: Review of Medical Physiology, 8th Ed. © by Lange Medical Books, Los Altos, CA, 1977.)

vasoconstriction. Blood flow to the myocardium is also reduced by coronary artery vasospasm and/or atherosclerosis.

## Total Peripheral Resistance

Total peripheral resistance is the other determinant of BP. There is a direct relationship between systemic blood pressure and TPR, so that the greater the TPR, the higher the contraction pressure that the heart needs in order to propel the blood throughout the circulatory system. The afterload (i.e., the pressure the heart must generate to overcome the resistance of the periphery) is influenced by several factors, including arterial wall diameter and blood viscosity.

Peripheral resistance is primarily influenced by alterations in arterial wall diameter. The walls of the large arteries contain elastic tissue, while the smaller arterioles have more smooth muscle. The smaller the diameter of the blood vessel, the greater the pressure required to circulate the blood. The arterioles are the major site of the resistance to blood flow, and small changes in their diameter produce large changes in blood pressure. Stimulation of autonomic nervous system receptors in the smooth muscles of arterioles produce vasoconstriction or vasodilation. Table 2.3 lists blood vessel responses when cholinergic or adrenergic receptors are stimulated. Other conditions that cause vasoconstriction include decreased local temperature and angiotension II in the blood. Elevated local temperature, hypoxia, and acidosis produce vasodilation.

Blood viscosity is reflected by the hematocrit, or the percent of red blood cells in the blood volume. The more viscous the blood (as in polycythemia) the greater the pressure needed to pump the blood through the arteries.

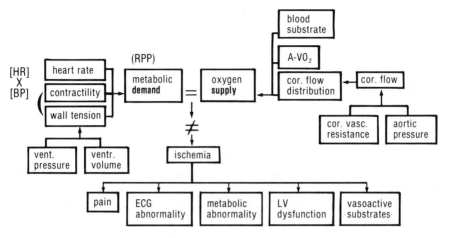

**Fig. 2.11** Illustration of the myocardial oxygen supply-demand relationship and the factors that influence the balance. An imbalance favoring demand results in clinical indications of ischemia. The rate-pressure product (RPP) reflects metabolic demand measured by the heart rate and blood pressure. (Adapted from Ellestad M: Stress Testing. Principles and Practice. 2nd Ed. FA Davis, Philadelphia, 1980.)

## Myocardial Oxygen Requirements

The amount of oxygen required by heart muscle when the body is at rest is determined by numerous factors. These include the amount of tension generated in the walls of the heart just prior to systolic ejection and the energy demands of a contraction. Both of these are clinically measured as the blood pressure. The heart rate, or frequency with which this pressure is generated, is also a major determinant of the myocardial oxygen requirement ($M\dot{V}O_2$). Basal metabolic requirements for cell life as well as the velocity of myocardial fiber shortening demand oxygen to a lesser degree. Factors influencing $M\dot{V}O_2$ are found on the left side of Figure 2.11.

A close approximation of myocardial oxygen consumption can be expressed as the product of heart rate and systolic blood pressure[4]; this index is called the rate-pressure product (RPP), or double product. An example of this relationship follows:

$$HR \times SBP = M\dot{V}O_2$$

$$70 \times 100 = 7000 \quad \text{(rest)}$$

$$200 \times 200 = 40,000 \text{ (vigorous exercise)}$$

As the RPP increases, myocardial oxygen requirements increase proportionately. If the coronary blood supply is unable to meet the increased oxygen demands, myocardial ischemia results and ECG changes and/or angina-pectoris may develop.

## PATHOPHYSIOLOGY

## Myocardial Ischemia

Oxygen delivery to the myocardium is limited by the supply of oxygen in the blood, ability of the coronary arteries to carry blood to myocardial cells, and the ability of the myocardium to extract oxygen from the blood. An abnormality in this transport and uptake system may cause the system to be inadequate to meet the metabolic demands of the myocardium. The resultant ischemia can present as one of a variety of symptoms signaling an unstable cardiac condition. Figure 2.11 illustrates the oxygen supply-demand relationship of the myocardium and the symptoms and consequences of an imbalance. Since the RPP is an index of myocardial oxygen demand, the onset of ischemia occurs at a consistent RPP.

Coronary blood supply to the myocardium can be limited by several conditions, including coronary artery disease, spasm, and myocardial infarction.

### Coronary Artery Disease

Coronary artery disease (CAD) is the most common cause of myocardial ischemia and is characterized by a buildup of atheromatous material (plaque) in the lumen of the coronary arteries.[3] The plaque may be found in a discrete lesion in a single artery or diffusely in any or all of the coronary arteries. The pathogenesis of CAD includes:

Injury to endothelial cell wall
Fibroblastic proliferation in the intima, causing it to thicken and thereby to narrow the arterial lumen
Accumulation of lipids at the junction of the arterial intima and media, further obstructing blood flow
Degeneration and hyalinization of atheromatous areas
Calcium deposition at edges of hyaline areas

This process of lumen narrowing usually takes decades, and symptoms typically do not appear until middle age when plaque formation begins to significantly narrow the lumen size and diminish blood flow.

Two major mechanisms appear to play a role in acute coronary vessel occlusion. In both, plaque may be present over years prior to an event such as an angina attack or myocardial infarction. Such an event can be precipitated by coronary vasospasm, characterized by sudden vasoconstriction triggered by unknown factors, possibly anxiety or cold air. The other possibility is clot formation, a complex interaction of factors, which is initiated by injury to endothelial cells or by plaque fracture.

The mechanism of blood clotting consists of a highly complex series of chemical reactions involving three phases of coagulation followed by a clot resolution phase.[5] Phase 1, the vascular phase, is characterized by two reactions to trauma: (1) local vasoconstriction and (2) mechanical pressure from blood leaking out to the tissue upon the injured vessel wall. Within seconds, phase 2 begins. This is the platelet phase, in which platelets become rapidly sticky in response to intimal damage. They adhere to collagen and vascular surfaces and aggregate. Blood flow slows down in response to platelet changes. Phase 3 is the coagulation phase in which plasma proteins interact to form prothrombin, which is converted to thrombin in the presence of a platelet factor. Thrombin formation also results from leakage of cell substances from damaged tissue. These plasma substances include fibrinogen, thromboplastin, and calcium. The next step in coagulation is fibrin formation from fibrinogen. This can only happen in the presence of thrombin. Fibrinogen molecules contain small fragments that interfere with thrombin activity, thus tending to limit the size of the clot. Large fragments, called *fibrin monomers,* combine, collect calcium, and become clots.

Clot resolution follows by interaction of fibrinolysin enzyme with fibrinogen to form fragments that have antithrombin action.

## Risk Factors for Coronary Artery Disease

Coronary artery disease has been implicated in one-third to one-half of all deaths in the United States. Over 4 million people alive today have suffered a myocardial infarction, a consequence of CAD. The high prevalence of the disease has been associated with numerous factors that place individuals at increased risk. Hypertension, hypercholesterolemia, and cigarette abuse are major risk factors for CAD, as identified by longitudinal epidemiologic studies, most notably the Framingham Study.[6]

Hypertension is typically defined as BP greater than 145/90 mmHg measured on three successive occasions, each one week apart. Fortunately, dietary, pharmacologic, exercise, and relaxation therapies have been successful in controlling high blood pressure.

Cessation of cigarette abuse can dramatically reduce the risk of CAD to half that of an individual who continues to smoke.[7] Much of the decrease in the incidence of CAD that has occurred during the past decade in the United States has been attributed to the reduction in smoking and to control of cholesterol.[8]

The major lipids found in the blood are cholesterol, triglycerides, and phospholipids. These lipids are carried in the blood by lipoproteins, each of which contains a relatively fixed proportion of the various lipids and has a predetermined carrier function. Both low-density and high-density lipoproteins (LDL and HDL, respectively) primarily carry cholesterol in the blood, LDL bringing it to cells and HDL carrying it away from cells. A decreased risk of CAD exists when total cholesterol is less than 200 mg/dL and the ratio of total cholesterol to HDL is less than 4.0. Very low density lipoproteins (VLDL) consist of the LDL remaining after the cholesterol component has been reduced and contain primarily triglyceride. Although elevated (fasting) triglyceride values are not considered risk factors for CAD, values greater than 250 mg/dL seem to be in an unhealthy range.[7]

Minor risk factors identified by results of the Framingham study are: diabetes mellitis, male sex, aging, obesity, sedentary life-style (less than 2,000 kcal utilized in leisure time activities per week), type A personality traits, and family history of CAD.[6] It has also been established that one myocardial infarction is a major risk factor for subsequent myocardial infarctions. It is important to note that patients who have peripheral vascular disease and present with histories of intermittent claudication, transient ischemic episodes, or cerebral vascular insufficiency have a high incidence of CAD as well. Risk factors that predispose an individual to coronary atherosclerosis may also contribute to the development of peripheral or cerebral artery atherosclerosis.

### Myocardial Infarction

There are three possible consequences of coronary atherosclerosis: angina pectoris, which is chest pain produced by the supply-demand imbalance of oxygen requirement in the myocardium (Ch. 4); myocardial infarction; and sudden death. Myocardial infarction occurs when blood flow is completely occluded in a coronary vessel and nutrient supply to a section of myocardium is blocked, which causes cells to die and tissue to become necrotic. The necrotic tissue is surrounded by a zone of cells that still receives some blood from other vessels but may be ischemic from loss of supply from one vessel. These cellular changes produce altered electrolyte flux across damaged membranes, and ECG patterns show specific changes indicating necrosis (ST segment elevation and Q waves) as well as zones of ischemia in surrounding tissue (ST segment depression) (Fig. 2.12).

When the coronary artery obstruction involves necrosis of the entire ventricular wall thickness, this is referred to as a transmural MI. Subendocardial infarcts are nontransmural and usually involve the inner one-third of the myocardial wall. Necrotic tissue gradually forms scar, over about 6 weeks. Before scar formation, the weakened area is susceptible to aneurysm development. Scarred tissue does not contribute to contractile force of wall motion during systole.[9]

## Congestive Heart Failure

When large sections of left ventricular wall are scarred from multiple myocardial infarctions or a massive area of infarct and prolonged ischemia, the ability of the wall to develop contractile force is seriously limited. The car-

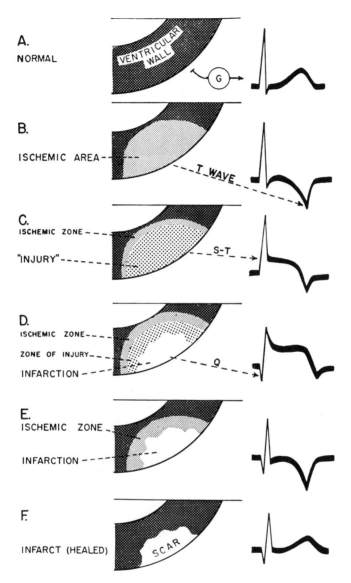

**Fig. 2.12** Electrocardiographic sequence of myocardial infarction. (**A**) A normal ECG pattern. (**B**) Ischemic area produces a sharply inverted T wave. (**C**) Myocardial hypoxia interferes with repolarization, producing an "injury" current and resulting displacement of the ST segment. (**D**) Q wave appears when ischemic area dies. (**E**) Injured area either remains ischemic or dies, returning ST segment to baseline. (**F**) Ischemic area returns to normal from collateral arterial blood supply, producing normal T wave. Only Q wave due to scar tissue remains. (Adapted from Rushmer R: Cardiovascular Dynamics. 4th Ed. WB Saunders, Philadelphia, 1976. Reprinted with permission from WB Saunders Co.)

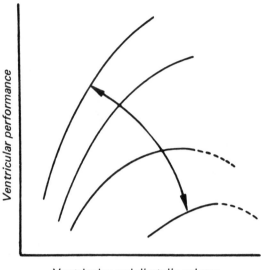

Ventricular end-diastolic volume

**Fig. 2.13** Effect of increasing end diastolic volume (EDV) on ventricular performance. (Adapted from Sokolow M, McIlroy M: Clinical Cardiology. © by Lange Medical Books, Los Altos, CA, 1981.)

diac output is diminished and the heart "fails" to accomplish its mechanical function. The results are minimal cardiac reserve, resulting in poor functional capacity, and low perfusion to peripheral tissues.[10] Congestive heart failure (CHF) can result from extensive loss of contractility of the myocardium. Heart muscle attempts to compensate for this decrease in inotropy by dilating its chambers, which should produce more wall tension (Frank-Starling law of the heart). At the point of dilation where muscle length is overstretched even less force is produced, and the ventricle has lost compliance as well as contractility (Fig. 2.13). The heart has less success than ever in emptying its contents and thus remains dilated (stretched). Resting end diastolic volume (EDV) is elevated, and the ejection fraction (EF), or percent of blood volume actually ejected, is low. Normally 60 to 80 percent of blood entering the ventricle is ejected, but in some patients with severe CHF, an EF of 10 to 15 percent can be indicative of poor ventricular function. Ejection fraction can be expressed by the following formula:

$$EF = (EDV - ESV)/EDV$$

where ESV = end systolic volume.

Other etiologies of CHF include cardiomyopathy, myocarditis, and mitral valve regurgitation. A clear sign of left ventricular CHF (LVCHF) is pulmonary edema, which will occur as a greater volume of blood remains in the ventricle, keeping internal chamber pressure too high. This in turn creates back pressure at the mitral valve, the left atrium, and thence the pulmonary circulation, causing breathlessness. Pressure in the pulmonary capillary system is an indirect measurement of left atrial pressure. When LVCHF causes left atrial pressure to increase, it is clinically measured by placing the transducer of the Swan-Ganz catheter in the pulmonary capillary wedge position (see Ch. 4). Elevated pressure in the pulmonary capillaries causes an increase in pulmonary artery pressure, and this creates stress on the right ventricle. Over time, the right ventricle can adjust to a higher pressure load by hypertrophy, but its capacity for this adaptation is more limited than that of the left ventricle, which is accustomed to high-pressure loads. It therefore begins the same changes in muscle length, dilation, and gradual loss of contractility as was seen on the left side. If right ventricular CHF (RVCHF) develops, the blood volume does not move briskly through the central circulation, and fluid accumulation begins to appear. Right ventricular CHF due to LVCHF is called *cor pulmonale*. Signs of RVCHF are jugular venous distention, peripheral edema, ascites, and cyanosis.

Pathologic conditions that obstruct the ventricular outflow tract also produce CHF due to the high internal ventricular pressures required to pump blood across the obstruction. As the heart muscle hypertrophies to generate a more forceful contraction, ventricular compliance decreases. Aortic stenosis and idiopathic hypertrophic subaortic stenosis can cause LVCHF in this way. Symptoms of breathlessness, fatigue, and chest pain are found. Right ventricular CHF can be caused by right ventricular outflow tract obstruction such as pulmonary valve stenosis or pulmonary hypertension.

Left heart failure is usually treated with diuretics to reduce blood volume and with digitalis to increase inotropy. Vasodilators such as prazosin and nifedipine have been used successfully in some patients to reduce afterload. When heart failure is compensated and subsymptomatic, exercise training can be used to improve function.

# EXERCISE PHYSIOLOGY

Tissue requirements for oxygen are increased by acute exercise. The cardiovascular system accommodates to this demand by increasing the cardiac output, which is distributed to active tissues by forceful pumping. This ability to increase cardiac output to meet the demands of exercise is called the cardiac reserve.[11] Both heart rate and stroke volume rise as components of cardiac reserve, the former linearly with increasing requirement (HR versus $\dot{V}O_2$) and the latter early in exercise and then leveling off to a plateau as work rate increases to maximum. Each of these has an enormous potential reserve (Table 2.4).

A reflection of the increase in force of contraction is the systolic blood

Table 2.4 Cardiovascular Responses to Maximal Exercise

| Variable | Rest | Maximal Exercise | Increase (%) |
|---|---|---|---|
| Heart rate | 65 beats/min | 195 beats/min | 300 |
| Stroke volume | 60 ml/beat | 120 ml/beat | 200 |
| Arteriovenous oxygen difference | 6 ml/100 ml | 18 ml/100 ml | 300 |
| Oxygen consumption | 250 ml/min | 4500 ml/min | 1800 |
| | 2.5 ml/kg/min | 63 ml/kg/min | |
| | 1 MET | 18 METs | |

pressure, which rises with rise in the cardiac output. The distribution of blood is altered by the peripheral demand of working muscle, which receives up to 85 percent of the total blood volume during vigorous exercise. Compared with resting muscle, which receives no more than 20 percent of the cardiac output, this is a major redistribution. The brain, heart, and lungs continue to receive the same percentage of the cardiac output at rest and during maximal exercise. The shift to working muscle occurs at the expense of the viscera and nonactive muscle.

Working muscle's extraction of oxygen from arterial blood, reflected by the arteriovenous oxygen difference $[C(a - \bar{v})O_2]$, is capable of rising by 300 percent from rest to vigorous exertion. This factor in combination with the cardiac reserve accounts for the 1,800 percent increase in total body oxygen consumption from basal resting state to maximal exercise (recall the Fick equation: $\dot{V}O_2 = \dot{Q} \times C(a - \bar{v})O_2$). Cardiac reserve is a consequence of several factors including sympathetic nerve impulses, circulating catecholamines, and the Frank-Starling mechanism. It is interesting to note that the Frank-Starling mechanism allows heart transplant recipients to increase their cardiac output at the initiation of exercise. Because of cardiac denervation in these patients, increases in chronotropy (heart rate) and inotropy (strength of contraction) from SNS stimulation are not possible. Rather, the initial elevation in cardiac output is due to the early increase in stroke volume, which is a result of greater preload from peripheral muscular contraction. As exercise continues in these subjects, subsequent increases in cardiac output can occur in response to circulating catecholamines.[2] Figure 2.14 illustrates cardiac responses to dynamic exercise in innervated and denervated hearts.

## Response to Static Exercise

Isometric contraction of any skeletal muscle to a force equal to or greater than 30 percent of the maximal voluntary contraction generates a pressor response. This level of contraction exerts an external pressure upon vessels located within muscle bellies and is sufficient to occlude smaller vessels leading to nutrient beds, thus rendering the oxygen supply to capillaries nonexistent. Isometric contractions are therefore supported by anaerobic

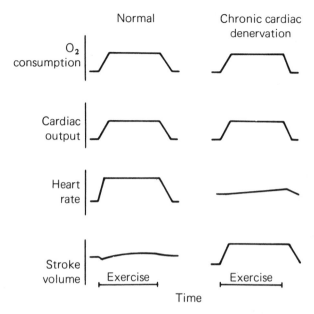

**Fig. 2.14** Cardiac responses to moderate supine exercise in humans. The responses labeled chronic cardiac denervation were obtained in patients with cardiac transplants. (Reproduced from Kent K & Cooper T: The denervated heart. N Engl J Med 291:1017, 1974.)

metabolism. The pressor response to isometric contractions relates to two mechanisms. One is the powerful activation of the adrenergic nervous system resulting in arteriolar vasoconstriction. The second reaction is owing to the mechanical squeeze of the contracting muscles. Both generate a significant increase in total peripheral resistance, with resultant increase in left ventricular afterload. The myocardium must generate a significantly higher force of contraction in the left ventricle to produce systolic ejection against a much higher pressure gradient in the arterial system. If isometric contractions were used as a training program, as in weight lifting, the afterloaded ventricle would have to respond with hypertrophy.

## Training and Detraining

The cardiovascular system is extremely versatile because it adjusts to the overall level of demand for metabolic support in a relatively short period of time. When the level of demand is elevated on a regular basis, as during a training program or with a change in occupation requiring habitual high levels of exertion previously untried, the cardiac output shows a much increased reserve. By the same token, with severe illness with enforced recumbency or with a period of sedentary behavior the cardiac reserve is appropriately

Table 2.5 Adaptation of Variables to Training and Detraining

| Variable | Detrained | Pretrained | Post-trained | Olympic Runner |
|---|---|---|---|---|
| Cardiovascular | | | | |
| HR[a] rest (beats/min) | 73 | 68 | 59 | 38 |
| HR peak ex (beats/min) | 150 | 185 | 183 | 174 |
| SV[a] rest (ml) | 55 | 65 | 80 | 125 |
| SV peak ex (ml) | 100 | 120 | 140 | 200 |
| $\dot{Q}$[a] rest (L/min) | 4.0 | 4.4 | 4.7 | 4.8 |
| $\dot{Q}$ peak ex (L/min) | 15 | 22.2 | 25.6 | 34.8 |
| Heart vol (ml) | 650 | 750 | 820 | 1200 |
| Blood vol (L) | 4.1 | 4.7 | 5.1 | 6.0 |
| SBP[a] rest (mmHg) | 140 | 135 | 130 | 120 |
| SBP peak ex (mmHg) | 210 | 210 | 205 | 210 |
| DBP[a] rest (mmHg) | 80 | 78 | 76 | 65 |
| DBP peak ex (mmHg) | 85 | 82 | 80 | 65 |
| Metabolic | | | | |
| $C(a - \bar{v})O_2$[a] rest | 6.0 | 6.0 | 6.0 | 6.0 |
| $C(a - \bar{v})O_2$ peak ex | 14.0 | 14.5 | 15.0 | 16.0 |
| $\dot{V}O_2$[a] rest (ml/kg/min) | 2.4 | 2.6 | 2.8 | 2.9 |
| $\dot{V}O_2$ peak ex (ml/kg/min) | 21 | 32.2 | 38.4 | 56 |
| Blood lactate rest | 10 | 10 | 10 | 10 |
| Blood lactate peak ex | 100 | 110 | 125 | 185 |

[a] HR, SV, $\dot{Q}$, SBP, DBP, $C(a - \bar{v})O_2$, and $\dot{V}O_2$ are, respectively, heart rate, stroke volume, cardiac output, systolic blood pressure, diastolic blood pressure, arteriovenous $O_2$ difference, and oxygen consumption.

reduced. Homeostatic mechanisms are constantly in play to keep the body systems attuned to the level of functional requirements.

In contrast to myocardial adjustments occurring in response to weight training, which increase the afterload, as mentioned above, aerobic training produces adjustments based on preloading the ventricle. Dynamic use of peripheral muscles promotes venous return and facilitates the thoracic pump to return the blood volume to the central circulation. The thoracic pump contributes significantly to the venous return by the creation of larger and larger negative pressures as breaths become deeper with increased exertion. This suction helps blood to return to the heart. In weight lifting the subject unconsciously holds his breath, which effectively creates a high intrathoracic pressure. The stability this affords him for lifting heavy loads facilitates even greater load carriage, but this high intrathoracic pressure causes obstruction to venous return, so that less blood volume passes through the cardiac chambers. With dynamic exercise, more blood volume passes through the chambers; this results in an adaptation in chamber size that is not simply dilation but creates a brisk stretch with each cardiac cycle. The contractile forces generated are enhanced, the ventricle wall may hypertrophy to a small degree, and there is a general strengthening effect on both ventricles. The training adaptations produced by this type of exercise (e.g., jogging, cycling, swimming) are summarized in the Table 2.5.

Further discussion of human response to acute and chronic exercise is found in chapter 5 and the exercise physiology references listed at the end of this chapter.

# REFERENCES

1. Netter F: The Ciba Collection of Medical Illustrations. The Heart, Vol. 5. Ciba-Geigy, West Caldwell, New Jersey. 1969.
2. Ganong W: Review of Medical Physiology. 8th Ed. Lange Medical Books, Los Altos, CA, 1977
3. Rushmer R: Cardiovascular Dynamics. 4th Ed. WB Saunders, Philadelphia 1976
4. Kitamaura R, Jorgensen C, Gobel F, et al: Hemodynamic correlates of myocardial oxygen consumption during Upright Exercise. J Appl Physiol 32:516, 1972
5. Moore W: Vascular Surgery. A Comprehensive Review. Grune & Stratton, Orlando, FL 1983
6. Kannel W, Gordon T (eds): The Framingham Study. National Institutes of Health Publication NIH 76-1083. U.S. Government Printing Office, Washington, 1976
7. Kannel W: Cardiovascular disease: a multifactorial problem (insights from the Framingham study). In Pollock M, Schmidt D (eds): Heart Disease and Rehabilitation. Houghton-Mifflin, Boston, 1979
8. Goldman L, Cook E: Decline of ischemic heart disease mortality rates: an analysis of the comparative effects of medical intervention and changes in lifestyle. Ann Intern Med 101:825, 1984
9. Sokolow M, McIlroy M: Clinical Cardiology. Lange Medical Books, Los Altos, CA, 1981
10. Berne R, Levy M: Cardiovascular Physiology. 3rd Ed. CV Mosby, St Louis, 1977
11. Astrand P, Rohdal, K: Textbook of Work Physiology. 3rd Ed. McGraw-Hill, New York, 1986

# PHYSICAL THERAPY EVALUATION

3

Patients present with, develop, or later complain of a variety of symptoms coincidental with their physical therapy treatments. It is certainly well understood that a variety of physical agents and exercise techniques used by physical therapists for a variety of indications result in cardiac, peripheral vascular, and pulmonary adjustments. In certain patients the stimulus that is presented by these treatments may be too stressful for appropriate accommodation of the patient's fragile physiologic mechanisms. Treatment decisions must therefore include determination of the appropriateness of a specific treatment and individualization of the dose of each component of the treatment. These decisions are based on the most complete understanding of the patient's pretreatment physiologic status. To be fully prepared to make these decisions, the chart review is an essential information resource.

In many patients with symptoms that may arise from cardiopulmonary problems, certain tests and procedures may have been performed that will shed light upon the patient's basic physiology. Not all tests are well understood, and the report of results in the medical record may be obscure. Also, certain tests have several names. We have selected the most commonly used name in our own experience for such tests. It is in part our intention to help interpret relevant test results in chart reports. From better comprehension of the chart data physical therapists can proceed to obtain their own data bases to supplement their ability to effectively plan treatment programs.

We believe that each patient interview should contain a number of common factors that are not symptom-specific and should also include some key questions that will shed light upon the specific symptom relevant to the patient (Table 3.1). Also there are a number of generic components to a physical therapist's evaluation (as presented in this chapter), which become more specific as specific symptoms are addressed. The following chapters discuss individual symptoms and provide those key questions to supplement

Table 3.1 Physical Therapy Interview

| Goals of the Interview | Ways to Achieve |
|---|---|
| Establish rapport | Facilitate patient comfort |
| Determine health belief | Explore patient's concept of responsibility for own health |
| Determine perception of symptom | See key questions |
| Determine perception of disease | Question the significance of the disease label |
| Determine patient's discharge needs | Assess motivation, cooperation |
| | Assess need for new therapies in new setting |
| Determine personal goals | Question premorbid desirable activities and explore patient's sense of quality of life |
| Determine previous activity and present functional level | Functional activity assessment |
| | Past work, social, leisure hobbies and activities of daily living |
| Determine family, household resources | Investigate family attitudes and availability |
| | Explore access to emergency medical system |
| | Evaluate ADL assistive devices, architectural features |
| Risk factor assessment | Cigarette use |
| | Environmental exposure to cigarettes and pollutants |
| | Coronary artery disease risk factor evaluation |
| | Genetic predisposition |
| | Anxiety disorder |
| Determine functional limitation | Mobility limitation |
| | Sleep patterns, eating ability, sexual activity |
| Determine medications | Have patient bring in drug containers |

the more general interview as well as the more specific evaluation tools or methods relevant to the individual symptom.

We split our generic evaluation into two important parts, the musculoskeletal and the cardiopulmonary evaluation. In this section we present a comprehensive list of those variables that could be included in a generic evaluation. Obviously, not all components of these evaluations need be performed in all patients. Any physical therapist is selective in the procedures used to evaluate a patient. In the chapters to follow we have discussed what we feel to be the most informative evaluation measurements for each symptom.

# MUSCULOSKELETAL EVALUATION

The components of the musculoskeletal evaluation are: (1) general range of motion; (2) general strength and endurance; (3) sensation; (4) balance/coordination; and (5) history or signs of trauma.

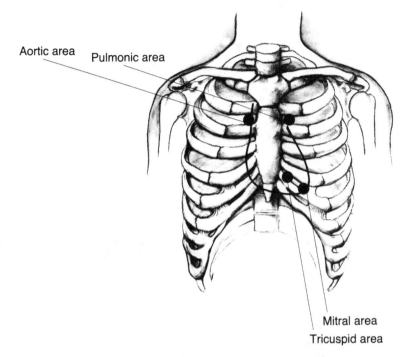

**Fig. 3.1** Areas to auscultate for sounds generated from the aortic, pulmonic, tricuspid, and mitral valves. In the normal heart the mitral area is the apical pulse point and the point of maximal impulse (PMI). (Reproduced from Bates B: A Guide to Physical Examination p. 125. JB Lippincott, Philadelphia, 1974.)

## CARDIOPULMONARY EVALUATION

The components of the cardiopulmonary evaluation are (1) inspection; (2) palpation; (3) percussion; (4) auscultation; and (5) assessment of vital signs.

## Inspection

The signs to look for in the preliminary inspection are:

1. Accessory muscle use in breathing
2. Symmetrical thoracic excursion
3. Paradoxical abdominal motion
4. Pursed-lips breathing
5. Spinal deformity
6. Cardiac apical pulsation (Fig. 3.1)
7. Patient color (pallor, red, blue)

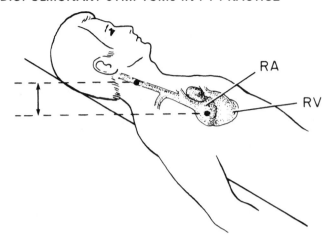

**Fig. 3.2** Examination of jugular venous pulse and estimation of venous pressure. RA-right atrium; RV-right ventricle. (Reproduced from Sokolow M, McIlroy M: Clinical Cardiology. p. 45 1981. © by Lange Medical Books, Los Altos, CA.)

8. Fingernail clubbing
9. Cyanosis of lips, nail beds
10. General health appearance (frail, cachectic)
11. Trophic changes of skin
12. Sternal scar, any other scar
13. Jugular vein distention (JVD) (Fig. 3.2)

## Palpation

The palpation procedure is as follows:

Place hand over cardiac apex position (fifth intercostal space) to feel for location of point of maximal impulse sensation (PMI).

Locate chest wall muscle trigger points. Apply pressure with heel of hand at sternal-costal joints to attempt to reproduce chest wall pain. Repeat over other painful sites.

Place thumbs over distal sternal-costal borders to measure distance of motion with deep inspiration and full expiration. Note asymmetry (Fig. 3.3).

Check for presence or absence of carotid, radial or brachial, femoral, popliteal, and tibial peripheral pulses.

Check for skin temperature, especially asymmetry and skin dampness, dryness

Check for pitting edema

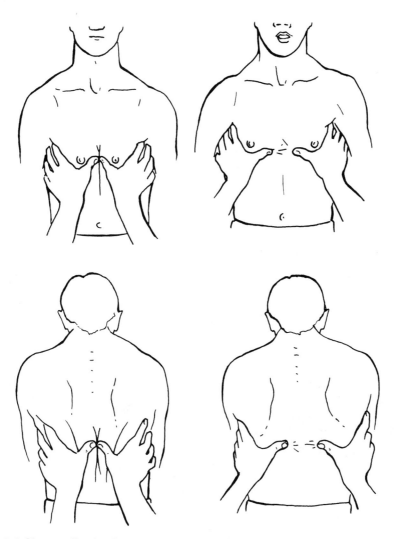

**Fig. 3.3** Chest wall palpation. (Reproduced from Cherniack RM, Cherniack L, Naimark A: Respiration in Health and Disease. p. 242. 2nd Ed. WB Saunders, Philadelphia, 1972. Reprinted with permission from WB Saunders Co.)

## Percussion

For evaluation by percussion, place a finger over the intercostal spaces at symmetrical lung segments from apex to base. Tap with the opposite finger over the finger at each site. Listen for different qualities of resonance.

## Auscultation

The auscultation procedure is as follows:

With diaphragm of stethoscope, listen for symmetrical breathsounds from apex to base.

With diaphragm of stethoscope placed at apex of heart, listen for presence of S1, S2 ("lub dub") sounds.

With bell of stethoscope placed at apex of heart listen for low-frequency S3, S4 sounds.

Combine auscultation of S1 and S2 with palpation of peripheral pulses.

## Vital Signs

### Heart Rate

By Palpation

Count number of beats in 10 seconds and multiply by 6 unless pulse is irregular, in which case count for full 60 seconds to get accurate heart rate.

By ECG Strip

If paper is marked in 3-second segments, count number of QRS complexes in 6 seconds and multiply by 10. If paper is not time-marked, use a rate stick: place arrow on the rate stick on a clear R-wave peak and count R waves according to the directions on the rate stick (can be 2 or 3). Read heart rate where the last R wave falls on the calibrated rate stick (Fig. 3.4).

An alternate method is to count time intervals on the ECG paper between two consecutive R waves (Fig. 3.5).

### Heart Rhythm

For an ECG rhythm strip:

1. Place bipolar electrodes (grounded), one negative, one positive, in position to pick up electrocardiogram with minimal muscle artifact.
2. Use either telemetry or hard wire.
3. Observe an ECG on oscilloscope or strip recorder over at least 30 seconds.
4. Note rhythm.

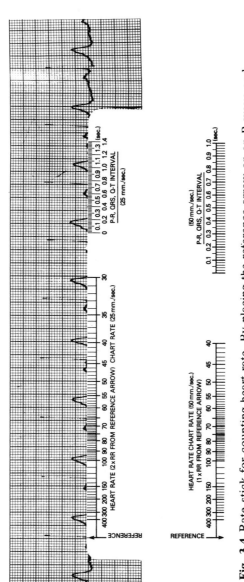

**Fig. 3.4** Rate stick for counting heart rate. By placing the reference arrow on an R wave and counting 2 R-R intervals, the rate is determined to be 67 beats per minute.

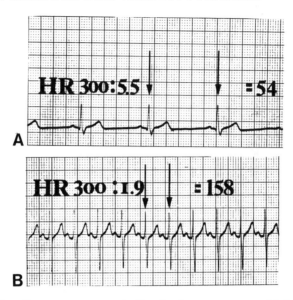

**Fig. 3.5 (A)** Two R waves are separated by five large squares and 2.5 small squares; the heart rate is therefore 300/5.5 = 54 beats per mintue. **(B)** Two R waves are separated by one large square and 4.5 small squares; therefore the heart rate is 300/1.9 = 158 beats per minute. (Reproduced from Thys D, Kaplan J: The ECG in Anesthesia and Critical Care. p. 12. Churchill Livingstone, New York, 1987.)

## Blood Pressure

The mercury manometer is the standard device used for blood pressure (BP) determination. An anaeroid gauge is also widely used but is more difficult to keep in calibration. The indirect method is based on Korotkoff sounds, which are created by the disturbance to blood flow when the external cuff occludes flow, then gradually permits flow to resume. Sound in the circulatory system depends upon turbulence of blood flow. Inflation of the cuff imposes a disturbance to blood flow which creates sound that is audible with a stethoscope.

The procedure for measuring BP is as follows:

1. Apply the cuff with the lower margin $2\frac{1}{2}$ cm above the antecubital space, the rubber bag over the inner aspect of the arm.
2. Place the stethoscope on the antecubital space over the palpable brachial artery.
3. Pump the pressure to a level approximately 30 mmHg above the patient's suspected systolic pressure or above the point at which the radial pulse disappears.
4. Release the pressure at a rate of 2 to 3 mmHg/sec. Faster or slower release will cause systematic error.

## Korotkoff Sounds

Korotkoff sounds become audible and pass through several phases.

Phase 1: The first appearance of a faint, clear tapping gradually increasing in intensity. This corresponds to first flow of blood through mostly occluded artery.

Phase 2: A murmur, or swishing sound, is heard, representing the major quantity of blood passing down the artery.

Phase 3: Sounds are crisper and increase in intensity as the artery continues to widen and allow more blood to flow.

Phase 4: A distinct abrupt muffling of sound occurs, with a soft blowing quality to the sound, at a point corresponding to the onset of laminar flow.

Phase 5: Sounds disappear as total blood flows in a laminar fashion through the artery no longer occluded by external pressure.

The systolic BP is recorded at phase 1 when the initial tapping sounds are heard for at least two beats. The diastolic BP is recorded at phase 4 or muffling. The American Heart Association recommends recording the diastolic BP at both phase 4 and 5. Usually phases 4 and 5 appear simultaneously, making the distinction difficult to appreciate.

## Manometer Readings

Current norms for sphygmomanometer readings are:

> Normotensive: SBP 110 to 130 mmHg
> DBP 60–80 mmHg
> Hypertensive: SBP 140 mmHg or higher
> DBP 90 or higher mmHg
> Hypotensive: SBP 90 mmHg or less
> DBP 60 mmHg or less[1]

## Respiratory Rate

> Observe breathing motion unobtrusively.
> Count one count for inspiratory and expiratory phase.
> Count for 10 seconds and multiply by 6.

## Temperature

Use oral thermometer for 1 minute; normal is 98.6°F or 37°C.

## Oxygen Saturation

Use ear or finger oximeter for reading in percent. Normal is between 95 and 100 percent.

### Cough (see Ch. 10)

Listen to Cough

> Sudden explosive onset?
> Audible sounds produced by secretions?
> Stridor (tracheal sound) present?
> Wheeze audible (bronchial sound)?

Observe Cough

> Inspiratory and expiratory movements
> Adequacy of inspiration preceding cough
> Spasmodic, long, ineffective, or crisp, forceful, short coughs, one or two at a time

Production of Sputum

> Characteristics of sputum
> Quantity, color, consistency, odor

### Functional Assessment

Specific Test Protocols

> Walk test: 12 (or 6) minutes
> Stairs
> Wheelchair propulsion (12 or 6 min)
> Ability to do all necessary activities of daily living (ADL)

Monitoring

Items to be monitored are heart rate, blood pressure, rating of perceived exertion (see Ch. 6), respiratory rate, and distance.

## REFERENCE

1. Gardner R: Arterial Blood Pressure Monitoring. A Summary and Manuscript. Dept of Medical Biophysics and Computing. University of Utah, LDS Hospital, Salt Lake City, June 1976

## SUGGESTED READINGS

Bouchier I, Morris JS (eds): Clinical Skills. WB Saunders, Philadelphia, 1976
Cash J (ed): Chest, Heart, and Vascular Disorders for Physiotherapists. Faber & Faber, London, 1975

Harvey A, Bordley J, Barondess J: Differential Diagnosis. The Interpretation of Clinical Evidence. Abridged 2nd Ed. WB Saunders, Philadelphia, 1972

Irwin S, Tecklin J: Cardiopulmonary Physical Therapy. CV Mosby, St. Louis, 1985

Petersdorf R, Adams R, Braunwald E, et al: Harrison's Principles of Internal Medicine. 10th Ed. McGraw-Hill, New York, 1983

Thompson J, Introduction to Physical Signs. Blackwell Scientific Publications, London, 1980

# CHEST PAIN

4

The diagnosis of angina pectoris, or chest pain due to cardiac muscle ischemia, may be relatively simple or extremely complex. Texts offering a comprehensive approach to differentiating sources of chest pain are readily available and routinely emphasize this point. For the purposes of this chapter an in-depth discussion of the clinical measurements, medical and surgical interventions, and physical therapy treatments associated with a diagnosis of angina pectoris will be presented. Other diagnoses of patients who present with chest pain are found in Table 4.1.

## CHART REVIEW

A medical record containing a history, physical examination, and results of diagnostic and laboratory tests can help the therapist determine the appropriate actions to take if chest pain occurs in a patient during treatment.

## Medical History

Much can be learned about the patient's symptom from an initial review of a comprehensive and detailed medical history.

Information regarding the "event" of anginal chest pain is typically presented in an organized and routine manner. An analysis of the following descriptors of chest pain can lead not only to the differential diagnosis but also to the appropriate actions to be taken in the clinic.

### Onset

The pain produced from angina usually occurs when the myocardial demands for oxygen supersede the oxygen supply available. Increases in heart rate, blood pressure, or both cause the heart to work harder and to need more oxygen. When there is an adequate myocardial oxygen delivery system, no symptoms are produced. However, in the presence of varying degrees of coronary artery obstruction, increases in heart rate or blood pressure, needed to accommodate necessary increases in cardiac output, may produce

**Table 4.1 Differential Diagnosis of Chest Pain**

| Possible causes | Possible Findings | Stimuli | Pathology |
|---|---|---|---|
| Myocardial ischemia | Pressure, ache, tightness, burning in midsternum, left shoulder, arm; diaphoresis; nausea; vomiting; ST-T wave changes; catheterization data show lesion | Exertion<br>Cold air<br>Smoking<br>Heavy meal<br>Fluid overload<br>Ventricular ectopy | Coronary artery disease<br>Coronary artery spasm |
| Inflammation | Auscultation of a friction rub; sharp pain, worsens with inspiration, improves with sitting | CABG<br>Acute MI | Pericarditis |
| Infection | Chest tightness with breathlessness; low grade fever; malaise; arthralgias | IV drug use<br>Microbes | Myocarditis<br>Endocarditis |
| Musculoskeletal | | | |
| Neck | Sharp pain with radiation to fingers; tingling; arthritic changes on x-ray | Neck motion<br>Posture | Degenerative joint disease |
| Sternocostal | Improves with stretching, with heat; arthritic changes on chest x-ray | Inspiration<br>Stretching<br>Local pressure to produce joint motion<br>Cough<br>Arm stretching | Degenerative joint disease |
| Post-coronary artery bypass graft | Feeling as if incision will separate; deep pain; sore | | |
| Pulmonary | Sharp, stabbing, pain; auscultate rub of lungs on pleura<br>Hemoptysis; breathlessness; cough; increased respiratory rate; increased heart rate; loss of consciousness; V/Q shows increased dead space | Deep breath<br>Prolonged bedrest<br>Recent MI<br>Recent surgery<br>Fracture of long bone<br>Atrial fibrillation | Pleurisy<br>Pulmonary embolus |
| Vascular | Searing; severe pain; sudden onset; decreased blood pressure | Trauma<br>Old age<br>Marfan's syndrome | Dissecting aneurysm |
| Referred pain | Burning pain; indigestion relieved by antacids<br>Belching | Heavy meal<br>Spicy food | Esophageal reflux<br>Hiatus hernia |
| Viral | Burning pain involving limited area over cutaneous distribution of nerve; skin lesions (vesicles) | Stress<br>Immunocompromise | Herpes zoster<br>Herpes simplex |
| Ventricular outflow tract obstruction | Angina pain; breathlessness; wide pulse pressure; hypertrophy of septum seen on echocardiogram; left ventricular hypertrophy on ECG | Exertion<br>Coronary artery disease | Idiopathic hypertrophic subaortic stenosis<br>Aortic stenosis<br>Mitral valve prolapse |

Table 4.2 Characteristics of Stable and Unstable Angina Pectoris

| Characteristic | Stable | Unstable |
|---|---|---|
| Frequency | Regular | Increasing per week/day/hour |
| Onset | Consistent and predictable | More easily induced; may change from only with exertion to during rest as well |
| | Occurs at same RPP[a] | Occurs at lower RPP than usual[a] |
| New onset | | Absent for a prolonged period and then returns |
| Location | Consistent | May become more variable with a spreading or changing radiation pattern |
| Relief | Consistent | Requires more sublingual nitroglycerin |
| Duration | Consistent | May take longer before relief |

RPP = rate-pressure product; see Chapter 2.

anginal chest pain. Consequently, classical "exertional" angina may result. Physical activities such as stair climbing, showering, lifting, pushing or carrying heavy objects, jogging, tennis, or weight lifting may bring on angina.

Blood pressure and heart rate are also elevated during times of anxiety or high emotion due to sympathetic nervous system activity. β-Adrenergic receptors in the ventricles cause direct increases in the force of myocardial contractility and hence greater oxygen requirements for sustained function. An increased oxygen demand in conditions of coronary artery disease (CAD) with limited oxygen supply can cause typical emotional stress-induced angina.

Additional settings that may precipitate anginal episodes due to alterations in blood pressure or heart rate are exposure to cold temperatures, exertion at high altitude, a large meal, anemia, dysrhythmias, aortic stenosis, and fever.

Occasionally, "rest" or Prinzmetal angina is described. This typically awakens the patient from sleep and is a result of coronary artery spasm, with or without concomitant coronary artery atherosclerosis.

Angina is described as stable or unstable. The former generally refers to a predictable, recognizable symptom relieved by a consistent action. Table 4.2 lists the characteristics of stable and unstable angina pectoris.

When chest pain is reproduced by direct palpation and pressure over the involved area, musculoskeletal causes are usually the source of the symptom. Angina pectoris is typically not related to inspiration or position. Chest pain that is affected by these actions may be due to pulmonary pathology.

### Relief

Generally, if exertion brings on anginal symptoms, rest will relieve the discomfort. Within moments of activity cessation, a decrease in intensity of the symptom is noticed, and complete disappearance of the complaint should occur within minutes. In some instances rest alone does not completely allow the myocardial oxygen demands to be met, and the assistance of pharmacologic agents such as sublingual nitroglycerin is warranted. Nitroglycerin reduces angina by causing an immediate reduction in venous return to the heart, thereby lowering preload and blood pressure. (The physiology of blood pressure is discussed in Chapter 2.) Nitroglycerin can also increase blood supply to the heart by coronary artery vasodilation. However, in long-standing CAD, atherosclerotic plaque may be calcified, which limits the vessel's ability to dilate.

Relief from chest pain occurring at rest usually requires administration of sublingual nitroglycerin. Removal of the anginal stimulus, such as emotional stress, cold temperature, or high altitude, may be sufficient to eliminate the symptom. In a stable angina pattern, rest and/or one to three sublingual nitroglycerin tablets typically and consistently provide symptom relief (Table 4.2).

When angina is due to fever, anemia, aortic stenosis, or dysrhythmias, treatment of chest pain is directed to correction of these conditions.

Substernal burning and indigestion may not be due to CAD. Relief of these symptoms with antacids indicates esophageal reflux as the probable cause of the symptom.

Chest pain from musculoskeletal causes such as sternocostal joint disease, nerve root compression, and sternal incisions may be relieved by analgesics, anti-inflammatories, and physical agents. Therapeutic exercise may also be helpful.

### Location

Although the pain of angina pectoris may be located anywhere from the waist up, it is classically substernal, with radiation down the left arm. Not infrequently, the pain radiates upward to the jaw and down the right arm or back between the shoulder blades. Patients have complained of symptoms in the throat, elbow, or wrist, and these may be unilateral or bilateral.

The reason for the variability of the radiation pattern is not well understood. A number of theories of referred pain have been postulated. Impulses generated from ischemic myocardium may converge on neurons traversed by peripheral (somatic) afferents entering at the same spinal level. Information is relayed to higher brain levels via spinal thalamic tracts and interpreted as a pain in the corresponding sensory efferent distribution, usually C8 to T5.[1,2]

All patients typically recognize the location of their own angina, as it frequently has the same presentation at each episode (Fig. 4.1).

### Quality

Words used to describe anginal symptoms are consistently recognizable as typical of the condition. Patients may describe a "squeezing," "tightening," or "pressure" in the chest. When symptoms radiate, there may be a complaint of "dryness in the throat," "heaviness of the arms," or a "dull ache

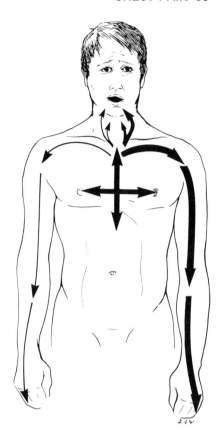

**Fig. 4.1** Principal areas of radiation of cardiac pain. (Adapted from Sokolow M, McIlroy M: Clinical Cardiology. © by Lange Medical Books, Los Altos, CA 1981.)

in the arm or jaw.'' Occasionally patients have a difficult time describing the symptom and are vague. ''Pain'' may not be described and patients may prefer to identify the sensation as a ''discomfort.'' Angina may be atypical and present as an ''inability to obtain a deep breath'' (in which case it may have a component of heart failure) or as abdominal discomfort or ''indigestion.'' It is important to note that a certain number of people with CAD will present with an anginal ''equivalent'' not associated with a chest discomfort. Frequently, patients with diabetes mellitus fit in this category and may only complain of shortness of breath or diaphoresis. It is in these individuals that interpretation of diagnostic tests is especially helpful. These tests are discussed later in this chapter.

## Intensity and Duration

In general, if the heart's demand for oxygen continues to be greater than the oxygen supply, chest pain will continue and intensify. Angina may proceed to infarction if the pain:

1. Continues to increase in intensity once the stimulus is removed
2. Requires more than three sublingual nitroglycerin tablets to gain relief
3. Lasts longer than 20 to 30 minutes

When myocardial infarction (MI) is suspected, the symptom is more likely to be described as "pain" and is associated with feelings of "impending doom." There is little correlation between severity of pain and the size of infarction. Diaphoresis, pallor, shortness of breath, nausea, and vomiting may be present with infarction but rarely with angina.

Chest pain lasting for a few seconds is unlikely to be cardiac in origin. Conversely, if it lasts for days without relief or intensification, the symptom is probably not due to myocardial ischemia.[3]

### Risk Factors for Coronary Artery Disease

Risk factors are routinely addressed in the medical history in an effort to identify candidates for early morbidity or mortality when CAD is suspected as the cause of chest pain. Does the patient have a smoking history? Is the patient's diet high in saturated fat and cholesterol? Does this patient have excessive emotional stresses at work or at home? Does the patient sit most of the day? Is leisure time spent exercising?

#### Implications for the Physical Therapist

If patient uses nitroglycerin, make sure he has fresh supply.

Check that the Physical Therapy Department's supply of nitroglycerin is fresh.

Look for exercise tolerance test in record to determine anginal threshold.

Be prepared to discuss risk factor modification with patient.

Verify that patient has not smoked a cigarette or eaten a large meal just prior to exercise.

## Physical Examination

Most of the information regarding a patient's CAD is obtained from a detailed history and tests. The physical examination may reveal very little.

### Physical Appearance

Patients experiencing angina pectoris may look normal and appear anxious. If cardiac output is compromised, patients may be pale, cyanotic, and weak.

### Vital Signs

#### Heart Rate

In general, there is very little unusual about the heart rate history in the symptom-free patient who is not taking any medication. The heart rate may be 60 to 100 beats per minute with or without pain. Sinus tachycardia (heart

**Table 4.3 Commonly Used Cardiopulmonary Medications—Effects on Heart Rate and Blood Pressure**

| Medication | Heart Rate | Blood Pressure |
|---|---|---|
| β-Adrenergic blockers | ↓ ↓ | ↓ |
| Methylxanthines | ↑ | ↑ |
| Calcium entry blockers | None or ↑ | ↓ |
| Sympathomimetics | ↑ or ↑ ↑ | ↑ |
| Parasympatholytics | ↑ or ↑ ↑ | ↑ |
| Diuretics | None or ↑ | ↓ |
| Angiotensin inhibitors | None or ↑ | ↓ |
| Vasodilators | None or ↑ | ↓ |
| Nitrates | Slight ↑ | ↓ |

rate 100 to 160 beats per minute) may be reported and can be due to a sympathetically mediated response to the emotional anxiety associated with chest pain. During an acute episode of cardiogenic chest pain the heart rate may be increased because of the pain or if exertion or a meal precipitated the symptom. As previously discussed, the increased myocardial oxygen demands stimulated by an increased heart rate may be greater than the available oxygen supply and will cause angina. Heart failure, due to a chronically ischemic myocardium and/or ventricular dilation, may present with sinus tachycardia as a compensatory mechanism to maintain cardiac output in the setting of a dropping blood pressure.

Subjects in excellent physical condition typically have slow heart rates (40 to 60 beats per minute), which in the absence of chest pain or symptoms are quite normal. Conversely, sinus bradycardia (heart rate less than 60 beats per minute) may be reported during cardiogenic chest pain. In addition to pharmacologic agents, a high vagal tone in this setting or an ischemic sinoatrial node may be responsible. Heart rates less than 50 to 60 beats per minute may be ineffective to sustain a normal cardiac output and may indicate a medical emergency.

It is important to note that various medications affect the resting heart rate and should be considered in interpreting this parameter (see Tables 4.3, 4.6, 5.4, and 5.5).

## Heart Rhythm

Heart rhythm may be reported as regular or irregular in the setting of chest pain. Many cardiac causes of chest pain can produce an irregular heart rhythm; however, it is unlikely that musculoskeletal conditions will alter cardiac conduction. Patients may describe "palpitations" or a "racing heart beat" or feel nothing abnormal. Any of these, as well as an irregular pulse, may indicate an irritable conduction system due to ischemia or conduction system disease. Electrocardiographic interpretation can shed more light on the nature of any pulse irregularities and is discussed in depth in Chapter 7.

## Blood Pressure

Blood pressure may be normal, but like the heart rate, it may be elevated if concomitant exertion, meal digestion, or anxiety is present. It is typical to find elevated blood pressures reported when acute myocardial infarction is suspected. Conversely, if heart failure is present, blood pressure may be low and indicative of a medical emergency. Table 4.3 lists medications that have an effect on resting blood pressure and should be considered when baseline data are reviewed. Blood pressure is not typically affected by cervical spine nerve root compression, but if there is arterial compression as well, it may be elevated. When chest pain is due to a dissecting aortic aneurysm, blood pressure drops as blood leaves the vascular compartment.

## Respiratory Rate

Respiratory rate is generally normal (14 to 16 breaths per minute) but may be elevated if components of stress, anxiety, or heart failure or lung disease are present. As mentioned previously, an increased respiratory rate may be characteristic of an individual's "atypical" angina. When chest pain is life-threatening, respirations may become irregular and shallow, indicating a medical emergency.

## Temperature

Temperature is usually normal in the patient with angina pectoris. However an acute MI can cause a low-grade fever due to inflammatory and reparative processes. Fever of any origin may produce a patient's typical angina because of the increased metabolic requirements. Cardiac or pleural inflammation causing chest pain may be associated with a fever.

## *Auscultation*

Interpretation of documented normal or abnormal heart or lung sounds can provide much insight into the cardiac and pulmonary systems. It is usually during exercise that the patient with a history of stable angina pectoris can have abnormal findings on cardiac auscultation.

## Heart Sounds

Normal heart sounds are generated primarily from valve closure and are labeled S1 and S2. These indicate the function of the atrioventricular valves (mitral and tricupsid) and the semilunar valves (aortic and pulmonary), respectively.

Murmurs are sounds generated by blood flow, typically across an incompetent valve. They are heard immediately before or after valve closure. Murmurs heard immediately after S1 are called systolic murmurs; diastolic murmurs occur after S2. Murmurs are best heard on the anatomic region associated with the valve generating the sound (see Fig. 3.1). Cardiac murmurs are not common findings in the patient with angina and/or CAD.

Complications of an acute MI can include rupture of an infarcted papillary muscle, rendering the mitral valve incompetent and regurgitant, or rupture of an infarcted interventricular septum. Both conditions can be associated with congestive heart failure (CHF) and pulmonary edema and produce a pansystolic (continuous) murmur.

Two additional heart sounds, S3 and S4, are seldom heard in normals but are very common in the patient with CAD. These sounds are usually best heard over the apex of the heart. Both S3 and S4 are generated by the influx of blood during early and late diastole, respectively. A decreased compliance of the walls of the ventricle when they are unable to stretch and accommodate the volume of blood entering the chamber can magnify the sounds, making them detectable with a stethoscope. When there is scar or hypokinesis in any area of ventricular muscle, the last bit of blood that enters the ventricles from atrial contraction may produce an augmented S4 heart sound heard immediately before S1.

Even more significant is the presence of an S3 which is heard shortly after S2, or semilunar valve closure. When an S3 is auscultated, it indicates a large area of noncompliant ventricular muscle since the sound is generated as soon as passive filling of the ventricle begins. Patients described as having an S3 are typically in heart failure and if not compensated pharmacologically, require medical attention. A comparably critical condition is the description of a "gallop" rhythm. This indicates the presence of both an S3 and an S4 (see Fig. 2.8).

## Breath Sounds

In general, the patient with cardiogenic chest pain has normal breath sounds. However, severe pain may cause the patient to avoid taking a deep breath. Muscular "splinting" as well as anxiety or depressed central nervous system (CNS) may reduce air movement in the bases of the lungs. If there is concomitant CHF and/or pulmonary edema, inspiratory rales may be described. If chest pain is caused by a pulmonary embolism, an expiratory wheeze, cough, and hemoptysis may appear (see Chapters 5 and 10.)

## Clinical Classification of Acute Myocardial Infarction

Patients suffering from an acute MI can be classified according to clinical findings indicating the presence or absence of left ventricular (LV) failure. Clinical signs of LV dysfunction, including dyspnea, inspiratory rales at the lung bases, and hypoxia, depend upon the size of the infarction, the elevation of LV filling pressure, and the extent to which cardiac output is reduced (see Table 4.4).

**Table 4.4 Clinical Classification of Acute Myocardial Infarction Determined by Repeated Examination of the Patient during the Course of the Illness**

Class 1: No clinical evidence of LV failure
Class 2: Mild to moderate LV failure. Rales lower one-third lung fields, possible altered S1 and S2, possible S3, arterial hypoxia
Class 3: Severe LV failure. Pulmonary edema
Class 4: Cardiogenic shock. Hypotension, tachycardia, mental obtundation, cool extremities, oliguria, hypoxia

(From Killip T, Kimball J: Treatment of MI in CCU. A 2-year experience with 250 patients. Am J Cardiol 20: 457, 1967.)

# Tests

Various tests are conducted to confirm the diagnosis of CAD as the cause of chest pain. Not all the following assessments are performed on every patient. Results of any one test can influence the physician's decision to perform subsequent evaluations. Test results may be very useful in helping the therapist assess the patient who complains of chest pain during treatment.

## *Laboratory Values*

### Stable, Chronic Patients

The patient in generally good health and with stable angina pectoris usually undergoes specific blood tests periodically. In reviewing these results, special note should be taken of the adequacy of the oxygen-carrying capacity of the blood, baseline electrolyte values, drug levels in the blood, and lipid and risk factor profile.

**Hemoglobin and Hematocrit.** The patient with stable angina pectoris may become symptomatic if the blood is unable to carry its normal amount of oxygen because the heart and lungs have to compensate and work harder to adequately deliver oxygen to body tissues. Blood tests that include hemoglobin levels and hematocrit can detect an anemia (see Appendix for normal values). In addition to dietary, genetic, neoplastic, and other organic anemias, depression of blood oxygen transport may be due to many pharmacologic agents, including quinidine, methyldopa, penicillin, and cytotoxic agents.

**Potassium Level.** It is important to consider potassium levels in the blood (see Appendix). Although CAD does not predispose a patient to electrolyte disturbances, pharmacologic interventions, specifically diuretics, may deplete potassium levels. Similarly, renal failure may cause abnormally high retention of potassium. Low potassium can predispose an individual to dysrhythmias such as ventricular ectopy, while elevated potassium can precipitate cardiac standstill. Either clinical manifestation can be accompanied by chest pain and lead to a medical emergency (see Ch. 7.)

**Drug Levels.** Cardiogenic chest pain can be precipitated by numerous dysrhythmias because coronary artery filling time and pressures are inadequate to perfuse the myocardium (see Ch. 7.) Several antiarrhythmic agents, such as quinidine, procainamide, and lidocaine, as well as digitalis, can induce dysrhythmias (see Table 7.2 and Appendix). A review of drug levels in the blood can alert the therapist to the potential exacerbation of symptoms if drugs are present above or below the therapeutic range.

**Lipids.** A close association has been found between elevated blood cholesterol values and the incidence of CAD. A patient whose diet is rich in saturated fat and cholesterol is at greater risk for CAD than one whose diet is mostly fish, poultry, fruit, and vegetables. Certain patients have an abnormal endogenous production of cholesterol or an abnormal transport of lipids in the bloodstream. Laboratory tests, including total cholesterol, high-density lipoprotein (HDL) and triglycerides can identify endogenous and exogenous sources of elevated blood lipids (see Appendix). The therapist should also be aware of blood glucose levels. High values may reflect diabetes mellitus, which is a risk factor for CAD.

## Unstable, Acutely Ill Patients

The patient who complains of prolonged chest pain, unrelieved by rest or nitroglycerin, and who carries the diagnosis of CAD or angina pectoris is typically evaluated for an MI. In addition to the previously mentioned laboratory tests, serum enzyme determinations are routinely performed. Blood gas analysis may also be performed.

**Serum Enzymes.** When myocardial cells are damaged, their cell membranes rupture, and enzymes normally found in high concentrations inside the cell are released into the bloodstream. Two of the most commonly measured enzymes are creatine phosphokinase (CPK) and lactic dehydrogenase (LDH) (see Appendix).

Elevations of CPK are typically seen in the first 4 to 8 hours after myocardial injury. Levels peak in 12 to 24 hours and are back to normal by about 48 hours after injury. The CPK isoenzyme specific to the myocardium is the MB band (that for brain is BB and for skeletal muscle is MM). The degrees of enzyme and isoenzyme elevation above normal have been correlated with the amount of damaged myocardium. This information can be useful to the therapist in planning the rate of progression in a therapeutic regimen for an acutely ill patient. Knowledge of peak CPK-MB elevations for patients with a history of MI can help the therapist to modify the therapeutic program according to the size of the infarction.

Other conditions that elevate CPK values include early successful reperfusion with fibrinolytic or thrombolytic therapy, as well as skeletal muscle trauma, such as that caused by open heart surgery or cardiopulmonary resuscitation (CPR).

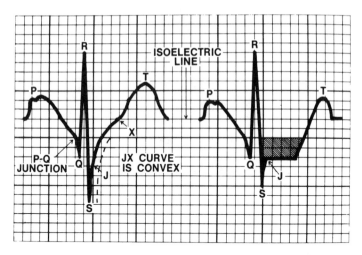

**Fig. 4.2** (Left): The normal exercise ECG complex. It can be noted that the PQ segment is deflected below the isoelectric line. This point is considered to be a baseline for determining ST segment abnormalities. (Right): A horizontal ST segment depression of 2.0 mm as measured from the PQ segment. (Reproduced from Ellestad M: Stress Testing. Principles and Practice. 2nd Ed. FA Davis, Philadelphia, 1980.)

Injured myocardial cells release LDH within 24 to 48 hours after injury. The enzyme reaches its peak elevation in 3 to 5 days and returns to normal by 7 to 10 days after injury. Several isoenzymes of LDH have been identified. Normally, LDH2 is greater than LDH1; however, when LDH1 becomes greater than LDH2, injury is specific for myocardial cells. Obtaining both CPK and LDH values ensures the ability to distinguish between a prolonged episode of angina pectoris and a myocardial infarction. It is believed that CPK-MB determinations are so specific for the diagnosis of an acute MI that LDH may no longer need to be routinely determined.

**Arterial Blood Gases.** Arterial blood gas (ABG) values are not routinely determined in the patient with CAD unless pulmonary function is compromised (see Ch. 5).

## Electrocardiogram

When a patient complains of chest pain that is thought to be due to coronary insufficiency, the resting 12-lead electrocardiogram (ECG) can be an invaluable evaluative tool. During conditions of myocardial ischemia, changes in the ST segment and T wave can be seen in the leads "viewing" the area of myocardium at risk. These would include T wave flattening, or inversion, and ST segment depression, with upsloping, downsloping, or horizontal take off from the J point (see Fig. 4.2). If immediate and adequate coronary blood flow is restored by rest or administration of sublingual nitroglycerin, the

ECG changes quickly return to normal. With myocardial injury, ST segments are elevated acutely in the leads "viewing" the injured portion of the heart. If the damage is subendocardial, the ECG returns to baseline in a few days. If the damage is transmural, the ST segments return to the isoelectric line and Q waves may appear in respective leads (see Fig. 2.12).

## Implications for Physical Therapy

The more extensive the ECG changes, the less the patient should be stressed.

Subendocardial MI may mean the infarction is incomplete and extending, and the patient should be less stressed.

### Exercise Electrocardiogram

While the resting 12-lead ECG yields valuable information in the diagnosis of an acute MI, a 12-lead ECG taken during exercise that provokes angina can effectively provide objective measurement of myocardial ischemia and can help to rule out other causes of chest pain. For example, as the exercise intensity on a treadmill or stationary bicycle increases, the cardiac output must increase to meet the oxygen demands of the subject's working skeletal muscles (see Ch. 5). To produce a greater cardiac output, the myocardium consumes more oxygen. In the presence of a hemodynamically significant coronary artery obstruction, this demand becomes too great, and several clinical responses may appear, including:

1. Changes in ST-T waves may occur on the ECG, with or without chest pain or an anginal equivalent. An exercise stress test is considered positive for ischemia when at least 1 mm of ST segment depression is maintained for 0.08 second (see Fig. 4.2).[4]

    The exercise test is interpreted as "equivocal" in cases in which the isoelectric line of the resting ECG is distorted by certain conditions, such as left bundle branch block. The ECG cannot verify the presence or absence of CAD in individuals with this finding.

2. A flat or hypotensive BP response to exercise may indicate left ventricular dysfunction. If coronary blood flow is inadequate to perfuse the left ventricle, the heart will not be able to generate sufficient pressure to perfuse the body. This abnormal blood pressure response to exercise may or may not be accompanied by symptoms including chest pain, lightheadedness, and shortness of breath. An exercise test may be stopped if a drop of 10 mmHg or more in systolic blood pressure is noted. Therapists should be alert to any acute drop in blood pressure in patients with known left ventricular dysfunction; it indicates that the work demand is too great for the heart (see Ch. 2).

3. Ventricular ectopic activity may be produced as the myocardium becomes ischemic. With increasing exercise work load, the ectopy is due

to cellular irritability resulting from hypoxia and may or may not be accompanied by chest pain or ST segment changes. With increasing ectopy there is a greater compromise of cardiac output, producing more symptoms of inadequate tissue oxygenation. An exercise test may be stopped when frequent unifocal premature ventricular contractions (PVCs), multifocal PVCs, or ventricular couplets appear. Dysrhythmias are discussed in further detail in Chapter 7. When life-threatening dysrhythmias of ventricular tachycardia or fibrillation are provoked, loss of consciousness may occur (see Chs. 7 and 9).

## Implications for Physical Therapy

The information obtained from an exercise test can be very valuable to the physical therapist in establishing objective guidelines for safe limits of activities. The amount of work a patient can perform on an exercise tolerance test (ETT) before symptoms or signs of myocardial ischemia appear can be represented by metabolic energy equivalents (METs); 1 MET equals 3.5 ml $O_2$/kg/min, which is the body's oxygen requirement at rest. Various exercise test protocols exist, and the work load at each stage of the test is quantifiable in terms of METs. Figure 4.3 gives examples of test protocols and MET estimates at each work load. The Bruce protocol is an exercise test commonly used for individuals with average or good exercise tolerance. It is not as informative for subjects who cannot complete more than one or two stages. Therefore, deconditioned or severely impaired subjects should be tested with a protocol that starts at a lower work load and has smaller work increments between stages, such as the Balke treadmill test.

Patients having sustained an acute MI can safely perform a low-level or modified exercise test as soon as 10 days after the acute event. The test is done to determine prognosis, efficacy of pharmacologic regimen, and exercise capacity. Patients who are at high risk for further cardiac morbidity of future mortality show the following clinical findings on low-level ETT[5]:

1. Onset of ECG changes (ST segment depression) at low workloads (less than 5 METs)
2. Onset of angina at low work loads (less than 5 METs)
3. Onset of significant ventricular ectopic activity (VEA) at low work loads (less than 5 METS)
4. Flat or hypotensive blood pressure response to increasing work loads

The oxygen demand ($\dot{V}O_2$) of many activities has been quantified in METs. For example, ascending a flight of stairs at a comfortable pace is approximately 5 METs (5 × resting $\dot{V}O_2$), walking 3 mi/hr on level ground is 2.5 METs, and values have also been determined for swimming, sweeping, etc (see Ch. 5 for detailed discussion of $\dot{V}O_2$ stress testing.)[6]

Although numerous tables have been published listing the MET value

| FUNCTIONAL CLASS | CLINICAL STATUS | O₂ REQUIREMENTS ml O₂/kg/min | STEP TEST NAGLE, BALKE, NAUGHTON 2 min stages 30 steps/min | TREADMILL TESTS BRUCE 3-min stages | KATTUS 3-min stages | BALKE % grade at 3.4 mph | BALKE % grade at 3 mph | BICYCLE ERGOMETER |
|---|---|---|---|---|---|---|---|---|
| NORMAL AND I | PHYSICALLY ACTIVE SUBJECTS | 56.0 | (Step height increased 4 cm q 2 min) | | | 26 | | For 70 kg body weight |
| | | 52.5 | | | mph %gr | 24 | | kgm/min |
| | | 49.0 | | mph %gr | 4 22 | 22 | | 1500 |
| | | 45.5 | Height (cm) | 4.2 16 | | 20 | | |
| | | 42.0 | 40 | | 4 18 | 18 | 22.5 | 1350 |
| | | 38.5 | 36 | | | 16 | 20.0 | 1200 |
| | SEDENTARY HEALTHY | 35.0 | 32 | 3.4 14 | 4 14 | 14 | 17.5 | 1050 |
| | | 31.5 | 28 | | | 12 | 15.0 | 900 |
| | | 28.0 | 24 | | 4 10 | 10 | 12.5 | 750 |
| | DISEASED, RECOVERED | 24.5 | 20 | 2.5 12 | 3 10 | 8 | 10.0 | |
| II | | 21.0 | 16 | | | 6 | 7.5 | 600 |
| | SYMPTOMATIC PATIENTS | 17.5 | 12 | 1.7 10 | 2 10 | 4 | 5.0 | 450 |
| | | 14.0 | 8 | | | 2 | 2.5 | 300 |
| III | | 10.5 | 4 | | | | 0.0 | 150 |
| | | 7.0 | | | | | | |
| IV | | 3.5 | | | | | | |

**Fig. 4.3** Oxygen requirements increase with work loads from bottom of chart to top in various exercise tests of the step, treadmill, and bicycle ergometer types. (Reproduced from American Heart Association, Committee on Exercise. Exercise Testing and Training of Apparently Healthy Individuals: A Handbook for Physicians. Dallas, 1972. By permission of the American Heart Association Inc.)

of activities, they are broad and variable and may be difficult to apply to activities performed in the Physical Therapy Department. The highest rate-pressure product (RPP) (Ch. 2) that a patient can safely achieve on the ETT may be a better and more individualized measurement for the therapist to use in establishing upper limits of exercise. Since angina is generally reproducible at the same RPP, activities or exercise performed in therapy should not exceed the RPP safely achieved on an ETT. For example, if a patient shows signs of myocardial ischemia on an ETT at an HR of 120 and an SBP of 150, then during physical therapy exercise this patient's RPP should not exceed 18,000. In fact, the therapist should allow the exercise response to be sufficiently below this "threshold" RPP to avoid appearance of the symptom and excessive risk. When the patient exercises on the *same* equipment on which the exercise test was performed, it is unnecessary to monitor the RPP as it is sufficient to keep the HR below the HR at which signs and symptoms of myocardial ischemia occurred. Upon completion of a safe exercise training program, a patient may be able to complete more work on a standard exercise test before the RPP threshold of symptoms or ECG changes appear.

Last, the rating of perceived exertion (RPE) is a scale developed by Gunnar Borg to enable patients to consistently rate their perception of the intensity of work. During physical therapy exercise the patient can report an RPE. This work level should be kept below the maximum safe RPE achieved during the ETT (Table 6.2).

There are textbooks addressing all aspects of exercise testing, including indications, protocols, interpretation, and application. The reader is encouraged to use these texts for further reference. Additional discussion on variations of exercise testing will be presented in Chapters 5, 6, and in case profiles.

### Radioisotope Scanning

The patient with suspected CAD may be unable to exercise because of physical limitations or severity of symptoms. Also, if the patient is able to exercise, the stress ECG may be unable to confirm the diagnosis of CAD owing to baseline ECG abnormalities or atypical angina. Under these conditions the utilization of radioisotope scanning, commonly with thallium 201 or technetium 99 pyrophosphate, with the patient at rest or exercising can add significant information regarding myocardial perfusion.

In general, radioisotope imaging can be used in two ways. First, scanning may be performed to study blood flow to the myocardium to determine hypoperfused regions; this is called *myocardial imaging*. Second, scanning of the intraventricular blood volume, or *blood pool imaging,* can be performed to determine wall motion abnormalities and to quantify left ventricular ejection fraction. In the latter determinations isotope imaging is synchronized or "gated" to the ECG.[7]

In the patient with a history of chest pain and with prior infarction, either myocardial imaging or blood pool imaging will help to locate and quantify infarct size but will yield little information regarding degree and distribution of coronary artery obstruction. Wall motion abnormalities are generally described as akinetic, hypokinetic, or dyskinetic, usually indicating scar, ischemia, or aneurysm, respectively. Ejection fractions can be quantified serially by blood pool imaging to monitor changes in left ventricular function in the days immediately after an acute infarction. Areas

EXERCISE          REST

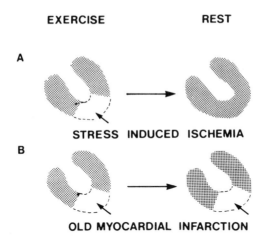

A

STRESS INDUCED ISCHEMIA

B

OLD MYOCARDIAL INFARCTION

**Fig. 4.4** Schematic representation of the changes in regional myocardial thallium 201 distribution from the early postexercise (Exercise) to the 4 to 5-hour delayed repeat images (Rest). As shown in (**A**), complete resolution of a defect is consistent with stress-induced ischemia. If, as shown under (**B**), the early postexercise defect remains completely unchanged on the delayed images, this most frequently is consistent with an old myocardial infarction. (Adapted from Wisenberg G, Schelbert H: Radionuclide Techniques in the Diagnosis of Cardiovascular Disease. Curr Prob Cardiol 4:7, 1979. Reproduced with permission.)

described initially as hypokinetic may return to normal motion or become akinetic.

For the patient with a history of chest pain but an equivocal exercise stress test result, thallium perfusion studies assist in diagnosing CAD. Thallium is injected during the last 30 to 60 seconds of peak exercise and scanned for myocardial uptake. The patient is reimaged after 2 to 4 hours of rest to detect changes in thallium uptake in areas initially hypoperfused. If the area remains hypoperfused, it is considered scar tissue. If thallium is reperfused in the area, the test confirms the inadequacy of coronary blood flow during increased myocardial oxygen demand. The larger this area of uptake, the larger the jeopardized area of myocardium. Occasionally in an exercise thallium test, the thallium portion indicates myocardial ischemia without simultaneous symptoms or ECG changes. This makes determination of safe exercise levels more complex as the thallium scan does not indicate the work load or RPP at which ischemia appears (Fig. 4.4).

More recently, thallium imaging studies have been used in combination with persantine for the latter's vasodilating effects. For patients who cannot exercise owing to physical limitations, administration of oral Persantine can stimulate coronary artery vasodilation. The relative hypoperfusion that is created through stenotic vessels can cause chest pain. Thallium imaging allows Persantine-induced ischemia to be detected and quantified. Since it is not an exercise test, no information is obtained regarding the functional level at which ischemia occurs.

## Implications for Physical Therapy

Nuclear imaging shows the extent of myocardial scarring and myocardial ischemia, which adds insight into how much cardiac reserve to expect for support of exercise.

## *Echocardiogram*

Echocardiography is generally performed to evaluate wall thickness and motion and valve function. Currently it plays only a minor role in the evaluation of the patient with chest pain due to CAD; however it is becoming more important owing to improved technology. The technique is noninvasive and is based on the finding that when sound waves of high frequency are directed into the body, they meet structures of varying densities and are reflected back into the transducer in an organized pattern. The ultrasound transducer is placed on the chest, and the beam is directed towards various portions of the heart. Any cardiac structure that is roughly perpendicular to the sound waves will be displayed on the oscilloscope.

Doppler echocardiography provides information on velocity of blood moving through cardiac chambers. Pressure gradients across heart valves can be calculated from Doppler studies to help quantify the severity of valvular disease. Color Doppler echocardiography allows a more accurate assessment of valve abnormalities, wall motion, ejection fraction, and chamber size.[8]

Two conditions related to CAD can be readily confirmed by echocardiography. In the setting of an ischemic, infarcted, or ruptured papillary muscle, mitral valve function may be compromised. The degree of hemodynamic impairment can be quantified with Doppler or color flow velocity measurements.

In the setting of a septal infarction and subsequent intraventricular septal defect, serial echocardiography can measure defect size. Again, if it is used in conjunction with flow velocity-detecting systems, the orifice size and flow direction can be measured.

Chest pain not due to CAD but occurring as a consequence of other cardiac conditions may be evaluated by echocardiography. These conditions include mitral valve prolapse, aortic stenosis, and idiopathic hypertrophic subaortic stenosis.

## Implications for Physical Therapy

Patients with wall motion abnormalities or low ejection fractions may have poor cardiac reserve and demonstrate exercise intolerance as fatigue and/or breathlessness.

Patients with large valve gradients may show signs of right heart failure, such as peripheral edema and cyanosis, or of left heart failure, such as rales, breathlessness, or cough.

Patients exhibiting mitral valve incompetence due to papillary muscle ischemia or infarction may become breathless before angina appears. Breathlessness is not an anginal equivalent but rather a consequence of pulmonary vascular congestion.

## Holter Monitor

The patient who complains of intermittent chest pain may also be evaluated with a continuous ambulatory ECG monitor. This "tape recording" apparatus is typically worn for 8 to 24 hours. Patients maintain a diary of symptoms and activities during the monitoring period. Although Holter monitors have been primarily used for dysrhythmia detection and quantification, recent advances in technology have made the correlation between ST segment changes detected by this device and CAD more accurate. Although ST segment depression has been found to coincide with reports of chest pain, the presence of symptoms without simultaneous Holter ECG changes does not rule out coronary insufficiency. Similarly, it is unclear how aggressive therapy should be when there is significant ST segment depression without symptoms. The therapist should be aware of the heart rate at which the patient complained of chest pain, as well as the heart rate when significant ST segment depression occurred. (see Chapter 7.)

## Coronary Angiography and Ventriculography

Cardiac catheterization is an invasive procedure used to define cardiac anatomy. A catheter is introduced into the heart, and a radiocontrast medium is injected into the coronary ostia. The medium can be traced fluoroscopically along the coronary artery tree so that partial and complete obstructions to flow can be quantified. Combinations of atherosclerotic plaque and spasm may limit coronary artery blood flow. The size of the vessel and its potential for coronary artery bypass graft (CABG) anastomosis are also assessed.

Ventriculography involves administration of radiocontrast medium into the myocardial chambers to assess the competence of cardiac valves, to identify wall motion abnormalities, and to quantify the ejection fraction (Fig. 4.5).

Hemodynamic measurements can also be obtained during the catheterization. Catheters with pressure transducers are threaded to each cardiac chamber and great vessel. Pressure waves are recorded in synchrony with ECG and phonocardiogram to assess the hemodynamic changes related to the cardiac cycle. Cardiac output can also be measured during the catheterization.[9]

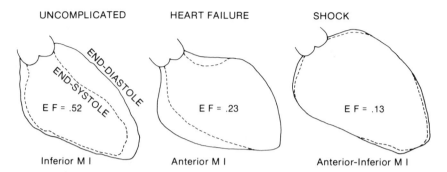

UNCOMPLICATED     HEART FAILURE     SHOCK

E F = .52     E F = .23     E F = .13

Inferior M I     Anterior M I     Anterior-Inferior M I

**Fig. 4.5** Diagrams of left ventricular angiograms of patients with acute myocardial infarction. The inferior infarction is associated with inferior wall hypokinesis and is clinically uncomplicated. Heart failure is associated with extensive anterior wall akinesis in the anterior infarction. The anterior-inferior infarction is complicated by shock resulting from the severe diffuse impairment of contractile function. Ejection fraction (EF) is progressively decreased with increasing involvement of left ventricular myocardium. (Reproduced from Amsterdam E, Wilmore J, DeMaria A: Exercise in Cardiovascular Health and Disease. Reprinted from Yorke Medical Books, New York. The Cahner's Publishing Company, a Division of Reed Publishing USA, 1977.)

## Implications for Physical Therapy

Patients with significant coronary artery lesions should be stress-tested to determine safe upper limits for exercise.

Patients with low cardiac outputs have decreased cardiac reserve.

### Chest X-ray

The patient with CAD does not routinely have a chest x-ray performed, but if heart failure is suspected or there are signs of left ventricular hypertrophy, a chest x-ray may be taken. (see Ch. 5.)

---

## MEDICAL-SURGICAL INTERVENTION

## Pharmacology

Medical therapy for coronary insufficiency focuses on the reduction of myocardial oxygen demand. Therefore, most of the pharmacologic agents used for the treatment of angina pectoris lower heart rate or blood pressure.

### Nitrate Therapy

Nitrate therapy is instituted to reduce ventricular preload by causing peripheral vasodilation. Nitrates act primarily on veins but may have some coronary artery dilating effects. Sublingual nitroglycerin is the drug of choice for immediate relief of coronary insufficiency. A patient may take three tablets spaced out over a 15- to 20-minute period to obtain relief of chest pain. If pain persists, additional pharmacologic intervention and evaluation may be needed. Patients should sit down when they take sublingual nitroglycerin. This will prevent traumatic injury in the event they become acutely orthostatic and fall as blood pressure drops. It is important to replace open bottles of nitroglycerin every 3 to 6 months because of the rapid deterioration of the compound. In addition to rapid-acting sublingual nitroglycerin, longer-acting nitrates are available (Table 4.5).

## β-Adrenergic Blocking Agents

β-Adrenergic blocking drugs reduce myocardial oxygen demands by decreasing the heart rate and the force of contraction in the resting or exercising heart. The less cardioselective agents in this group, (e.g., propranolol) may also induce bronchospasm and need to be used cautiously with certain patients (Tables 4.6 and 4.7).

Patients with moderate to severely depressed left ventricular function are rarely treated with β-blocker therapy since the negative inotropic effect worsens this condition. Beta blockers have been well documented to decrease the risk of a second MI if they are prescribed early after the first such attack. In addition to the above actions, β blockers have antiarrhythmic properties (see Table 7.2).

## Calcium Channel Blocking Agents (Calcium Antagonists)

Calcium channel blocking agents primarily act to decrease myocardial oxygen demand by lowering blood pressure. The blood pressure components affected are contractile force and afterload. Calcium entry into cardiac and arterial smooth muscle cells is blocked by these drugs. This reduces the length and degree of excitation coupling of myofilaments, inducing coronary and peripheral vasodilation. These drugs are particularly effective in reducing coronary artery spasm (see Tables 4.6 and 4.7). Verapamil, one of three widely used agents, also has antiarrhythmic actions and is often used in the management of supraventricular tachycardia (see Table 7.2).

## Antihypertensive Therapy

Drug therapy to reduce blood pressure is directed at alterations in the hemodynamic determinants of blood pressure. As discussed in Chapter 2, these include preload, force of contraction, and afterload. For purposes of simplification, the authors have addressed these drugs according to their primary antihypertensive effect. The reader should be cautioned that rarely do any of these drugs affect one component of blood pressure without causing alterations in another.

**Table 4.5 Characteristics of Nitrates**[a]

| Medication | Preparations | Onset of Action[b] (Minutes) | Peak Action (Minutes) | Duration |
|---|---|---|---|---|
| Nitroglycerin | Tablets for sublingual use | 2–5 | 4–8 | 10–30 min |
| Nitrostat | Sustained release capsule | 20–45 | 45–120 | 2–6 hours |
| Nitrobid | Ointment | 15–60 | 30–120 | 2–8 hours |
| (sublingual | Intravenous | | | |
| nitroglycerin) | Intermittent bolus | | | 3–5 min |
| | Continuous infusion | | | Continuous |
| Isosorbide dinitrate | Tablet for sublingual use | 5–20 | 15–60 | 45–120 min |
| Isordil | Oral or chewable tablet | 15–45 | 45–120 | 2–6 hours |
| Sorbitrate | Sustained release capsule | 15–45 | 45–120 | 10–12 hours |
| Nitroglycerine discs | 5–20 cm² disc | 30–60 | 60–180 | Up to 24 hours |
| Nitrodisc | | | | |
| Nitro-dur | | | | |
| Transderm-nitro | | | | |

[a] Side effects include headache, hypotension, reflex tachycardia, nausea, flushing of skin, throbbing of head and neck, palpitations.
[b] Primary action of nitrates is to reduce BP by lowering preload.
(Adapted from Ice D: Cardiovascular Medications. Phys Ther 65 (12):55, 1985.)

**Table 4.6 Common Medications Used in the Treatment of Myocardial Ischemia[a]**

| β Adrenergic Blockers | Calcium Entry Blockers | Diuretics | Antihypertensives |
|---|---|---|---|
| Propranolol hydrochloride (Inderal) | Nifedipine (Procardia) | Thiazides: Hydrochlorothiazide (Esidrex, Oretic, Hydrodiuril) | Sympathetic depressants: Reserpine (Serpasil) |
| Atenolol[b] (Tenormin) | Diltiazem (Cardizem) | Chlorothiazide (Diuril) | Methyldopa (Aldomet) |
| Metropolol[b] (Lopressor) | Verapamil (Isoptin, Calan) | Loop: Furosemide (Lasix) (Bumex) | Guanethidine: (Ismelin) |
| Nadolol (Corgard) | | Potassium-sparing: Spirinolactone (Aldactone) | Angiotensin II inhibitor Captopril (Capoten) |
| Pindolol (Visken) | | | Vasodilators: Nitrates |
| Timolol (Blocadren) | | | Prazosin (Minipres) |
| | | | Hydralazine (Apresoline) |

[a] A large selection of combinations of these drugs is available.
[b] Cardioselective

**Table 4.7 Primary Action and Side Effects of Medications Used to Lower Myocardial Oxygen Consumption**

| Medication | Primary Action | Side Effects |
|---|---|---|
| β-Adrenergic blocker | Decrease inotropy | Bronchospasm, CHF, hypotension, Raynaud's, worsening claudication |
| | Decrease resting and exercise HR | |
| Calcium entry blocker | Vasodilator (arterial) | Headache, hypotension, leg edema (nifedipine), digital dysthesias |
| | Reduce BP by decreasing afterload and reducing inotropy | |
| Nitrates | Vasodilation (venous) | Headache, hypotension |
| | Reduce BP by decreasing preload | |
| Antihypertensives | | |
| Loop diuretics and Thiazides | Reduce BP by decreasing preload | Electrolyte disturbance (decreased potassium), dryness of mouth, thirst |
| Potassium-sparing diuretics | Reduce BP by decreasing preload | Increased potassium, gynecomastia |
| Sympathetic depressants | Reduce inotropy | Postural hypotension, sodium and fluid retention, skeletal muscle weakness |
| | | Fainting, encephalopathy |
| Angiotensin II inhibitors | Reduce BP by decreasing afterload | Headache, sodium and fluid retention, gastrointestinal distress |
| Prazosin | Reduce BP by decreasing afterload | |

## Preload Reduction

Preload is reduced by nitrate therapy, as already discussed, as well as by diuretic therapy. The latter's effect is due to its action on kidney function by increasing sodium and water excretion. In addition to reduction of salt intake to lower water retention, diuretics are the mainstay of antihypertensive therapy (Tables 4.6 and 4.7).

## Reduction of Force of Contraction

β-Adrenergic blockers and calcium channel blockers can lower blood pressures by depressing inotropy. Other pharmacologic agents depress the sympathetic nervous system by action on postganglionic nerve endings, causing reduction in blood pressure; reserpine and guanethidine are such agents.

## Afterload Reduction

Calcium channel blockers lower blood pressure by relaxation of arterial smooth muscle. Nitrates also act on afterload to a slight degree. Other agents that have direct vasodilating effects include hydralazine and prazosin; however both may cause myocardial oxygen consumption to increase by elevating heart rate and/or contractile force. The formation of angiotension II, a potent vasoconstrictor, can be inhibited by captopril, thereby reversing elevation in peripheral pressure.

## *Antiarrhythmic Therapy*

Numerous drugs are used either acutely or in long-term management of arrhythmias. Table 4.8 lists first- and second-choice drugs used in the management of acute MI. A description of these drugs can be found in Chapter 7.

Ischemia-induced chest pain can cause an irregular heart beat warranting pharmacologic intervention. An irregular heart beat can cause chest pain related to decreased coronary artery perfusion time and volume, for example, a supraventricular tachycardia. Additional symptoms such as lightheadedness or loss of consciousness can accompany dysrhythmias. Chapters 8 and 9 discuss pharmacologic management of these symptoms.

## *Drug Management of Coronary Thrombosis*

Advances in this field of pharmacologic intervention for chest pain management have ranged from chronic outpatient anticoagulation and antiplatelet therapy to dramatic clot lysis during acute myocardial insufficiency. A serious limitation to the use of these agents is the risk of bleeding. However, since clot is frequently visualized when angina occurs during cardiac catheterization procedures, numerous physicians routinely prescribe chronic therapy to reduce clot formation.[4]

Table 4.8  Management of Dysrhythmias in Acute Myocardial Infarction

| Dysrhythmia | First choice | Second choice |
|---|---|---|
| Premature atrial complexes | Digitalis | Quinidine |
| Paroxysmal atrial tachycardia | Verapamil | Digitalis |
| Atrial fibrillation | Digitalis | Precordial dc shock |
| Atrial flutter | Digitalis | Precordial dc shock |
| Paroxysmal junctional tachycardia | Digitalis | Precordial dc shock |
| Premature ventricular complexes | Lidocaine | Quinidine<br>Procainamide<br>Phenytoin |
| Ventricular tachycardia | Precordial dc shock | Lidocaine<br>Quinidine<br>Procainamide<br>Phenytoin |
| Ventricular fibrillation | Precordial dc shock | CPR<br>Intubation and<br>    ventilatory support |

(Modified from Sokolow M, McIlroy M: Clinical Cardiology. © by Lange Medical Books, Los Altos CA, 1981.)

## Fibrinolytic and Thrombolytic Agents

The ideal drug for clot lysis necessary to preserve ischemic myocardium is not yet decided. Numerous clinical trials in this country and abroad are being run to investigate the efficacy of streptokinase, urokinase, and tissue plasminogen activator (TPA) administration during acute MI. Dosages and routes of administration have included bolus or slow-drip intravenous or intracoronary injection or infusion. Uncertainty also exists regarding how long chronic anticoagulation therapy should be continued.

## Anticoagulation Therapy

Patients with acute coronary insufficiency and MI receive heparin intramuscularly, intravenously, or subcutaneously to minimize further clot formation. Patients who received fibrinolytic or thrombolytic agents (discussed above), may also be maintained on heparin therapy. In general, the dose is adjusted to prolong clotting time, bleeding time, and prothrombin time and to decrease thromboplastin genesis. To maintain a level of anticoagulation in patients who are at risk for continued clot formation, such as those with restricted activity, those with left ventricular dysfunction and aneurysm, or those in atrial fibrillation, coumadin therapy may be instituted. Coumadin can be taken orally and acts as a prothrombin depressant. Patients taking coumadin have their prothrombin time checked regularly to measure the effectiveness of the drug. If the clotting time is excessive, patients may bleed too easily, and their coumadin dose is lowered.

**Antiplatelet Therapy.** Two other drugs used in the management of chronic coronary heart disease are aspirin and Persantine. Both these agents interfere with platelet aggregation and clot formation. It is believed that this therapy works as a protection against coronary artery obstruction.

**N-3 Fatty Acids.** Investigations examining the benefits of N-3 fatty acids (fish oils) in CAD are currently underway. It is believed that these substances may protect patients from coronary artery occlusion in two ways: (1) inhibition of platelet-aggregating substances in the blood (thromboxane 2); and (2) stimulation of vasodilating and anti-platelet-aggregating substances in the blood (prostacyclins).

**Implications for Physical Therapy**

In patients taking anticlotting drugs, check for hematoma, nose bleed, or other sites of bleeding. Protect from trauma.

Check laboratory values in patient chart for bleeding parameters to assess degree of anticoagulation.

## Lipid-Lowering Agents

Pharmacologic agents used in the treatment of hyperlipidemia are becoming more common, as dietary modification alone is not always successful in altering lipid levels. Unfortunately, some of these drugs lower total cholesterol at the expense of HDL-cholesterol. Also, side effects, including constipation, heartburn, and itching, may be intolerable, forcing patients to discontinue therapy. At present a combination of aerobic exercise and diet is the recommended therapy used to improve a lipid profile unless a genetic hyperlipidemia exists. Commonly used drugs are cholestyramine (Questran), lovastatin (Mevlocor), gemfibrizol (Lopid), colestipol (Colestid), and nicotinic acid.

## Antiinflammatory Agents

Pericarditis can be a sequel to an acute MI or a CABG. Signs of pericarditis include positional and inspiratory chest pain, pericardial friction rub, chronic ST segment elevations, and fever. Indocin (indomethacin) an anti-inflammatory agent, may be used short-term to treat this. Caution is needed with this agent since it can cause coronary artery constriction. A low-grade fever after an acute MI rarely requires an anti-inflammatory drug as it is a sign of the inflammatory response to myocardial necrosis.

# Rehabilitation

Rehabilitation of the patient with angina pectoris is directed towards preventing the symptom and maximizing patient function. The definition of rehabilitation of coronary patients according to the World Health Organization is: "The sum of activities required to insure them the best possible physical, mental, and social conditions, so that they may, by their own efforts, regain as normal as possible a place in the community and lead an active, productive life.''[10] This can be achieved through emotional support, education, and exercise training. The reader is encouraged to review references listed at the end of this chapter for an in-depth discussion of the rehabilitation process.

## Emotional Support

Denial of the existence of CAD, a classic response in this population, places the patient at great risk and causes tremendous stress to social support systems. The diagnosis can be extremely frightening to the patient, leading to overt denial. A patient may avoid using the words ''heart attack'' or may discuss the MI as if it had happened to someone else. Conversely, the fear of pain and of death from CAD can ''cripple'' patients, preventing them from functioning even within physiologic limitations imposed by the disease. Families may overprotect patients with CAD because they mistrust the patient's judgment. They may be so frightened themselves that they severely restrict the patient's activities. Supportive health care providers can facilitate the patient and family's adjustment and acceptance of the diagnosis. Participation in group activities with patients with similar symptoms and opportunities to verbalize these fears can ease this process.

Patients who sustain an acute MI require tremendous emotional support in the initial days after the event. Psychopharmacologic therapy may be appropriate during this time.

Once the acute reactions of denial, anger, and depression pass, patients and families need continued emotional support to help them accept the implications of the acute event. The patient learns to accept responsibility and control of the recovery process in order to ensure long-term life-style modifications and compliance with the healthful interventions necessary for future wellness. Ways to facilitate emotional adjustment include:

Frequently reassure the patient and family and provide them with simple explanations.

Give realistic responses to questions from patients and families.

Perform activities that the patient fears in order to build confidence during the convalescent phase.

Give information regarding activity limitations, activity progression, warning signs of myocardial injury, and drugs.

Support the patient through the difficult time of trying to change addictive behaviors such as smoking, dietary indiscretion, and inappropriate stress reactions.

## Educational Support

An understanding of the CAD process, including its etiology and its exacerbation of symptoms, can help both the patient and family become less fearful of the symptom and more responsible for its prevention. It is un-

Table 4.9 Risk Factors for CAD and Strategies for Modification

| Risk Factor | Strategy for Modification |
|---|---|
| MAJOR RISK FACTORS: | |
| High blood pressure | Medication |
| | Exercise |
| | Behavior modification: relaxation techniques, dietary restrictions (e.g., salt, alcohol) |
| Cigarette abuse | Behavioral modification: group therapy, hypnosis, participation in community programs |
| | Education series: breathing techniques, benefits of quitting |
| High cholesterol | Diet modification (e.g., low saturated fat, low cholesterol) |
| | Medication |
| | Exercise |
| MINOR RISK FACTORS: | |
| Diabetes mellitus | Diet control |
| | Medication |
| | Aerobic exercise |
| Sedentary life-style | Exercise programs: group or individual |
| | Increase leisure time activities |
| Obesity | Weight control |
| | Exercise |
| | Behavior modification: group programs |
| Type A personality | Behavior modification: group programs, exercise programs |
| | Education: classes, literature |
| NONMODIFIABLE RISK FACTORS: | |
| Aging | |
| Positive family history | |
| Male gender | |

certain how much patients learn during the first few weeks after an acute MI because of the emotional trauma of the event. Education should be reinforced throughout the hospitalization period by repetition of information and by providing much written material. Key areas to emphasize include:

Recognition of settings that trigger symptoms of ischemia and the appropriate actions to take

Drug information, including action, dose, frequency

Progressive activity for home including self-monitoring of pulse and RPE

Introduction to CAD and risk factors

Several weeks after an acute event, patients may begin to recognize their responsibility in the management of this disease. Health care providers can educate patients about risk factors of CAD and recommend strategies for modification of these factors. See Table 4.9.

Written material, class lectures, and group support all offer starting points for patients to implement new behaviors. Patients can be taught to recognize factors in their behavior that may make them become noncom-

Table 4.10 Benefits of Aerobic Training in CAD Patients

Improved physical working capacity
    Able to endure at a higher exertional level for a longer period of time
    Able to perform more work at lower heart rate
    Able to perform more work at lower blood pressure
    Able to perform more work at lower rate-pressure product
Improved lactate tolerance
Improved $C(a - \bar{v})O_2$ difference, maximum and submaximum work
Higher maximum $\dot{V}O_2$
Higher resting and exercise stroke volume
Higher HDL
Higher maximum cardiac output
Higher maximum minute ventilation
Higher efficiency of breathing
Lower resting heart rate
Lower resting blood pressure
Lower percent body fat
Less neurohumoral over-reactivity
Possible benefits:
    Joie de vivre
    Increased coronary collateral circulation
    Increased diameter of coronary arteries
    Regression of coronary atherosclerosis
    Less platelet stickiness

pliant with their wellness program. An ongoing education series can provide both current information regarding CAD management and continued encouragement of the group effort to comply with new behaviors.

## Exercise Training

Participation in an exercise training program can improve the patient's physical and emotional acceptance of CAD. Although it has not been proved, there is also a possibility that aerobic exercise may facilitate disease regression.

### Physical Benefits

The physiologic benefits that can be achieved with an aerobic exercise program generally reflect increases in the patient's physical working capacity. Table 4.10 lists some of the benefits of conditioning in patients with CAD.

Some studies have shown that activities that utilize approximately 2,000 kcal/week will prevent CAD and its progression, if already present, and promote longevity.[11] The types of exercise necessary to obtain these effects are those that use large muscle groups in reciprocal motions, such as walking, jogging, swimming, rowing, cycling, and cross-country skiing.

Hagberg and associates have demonstrated that when patients with CAD exercise at 90 percent of their maximum safe heart rate on a regular basis for 1 year, stroke volume during exercise can increase by 18 percent which suggests central cardiac improvements in addition to peripheral ad-

**Table 4.11 NYHA Functional and Therapeutic Classification of Heart Disease**

Functional Capacity:

Class   I: No limitation of physical activity. Ordinary physical activity does not cause undue fatigue, palpitation, dyspnea, or anginal pain.

Class  II: Slight limitation of physical activity. Comfortable at rest, but ordinary physical activity results in fatigue, palpitation, dyspnea, or anginal pain.

Class III: Marked limitation of physical activity. Comfortable at rest, but less than ordinary activity causes fatigue, palpitation, dyspnea, or anginal pain.

Class IV: Unable to carry on any physical activity without discomfort. Symptoms of cardiac insufficiency or of the anginal syndrome may be present even at rest. If any physical activity is undertaken, discomfort is increased.

Therapeutic Classification:

Class A: Physical activity need not be restricted.

Class B: Ordinary physical activity need not be restricted, but unusually severe or competitive efforts should be avoided.

Class C: Ordinary physical activity should be moderately restricted, and more strenuous efforts should be discontinued.

Class D: Ordinary physical activity should be markedly restricted.

Class E: Patient should be at complete rest, confined to bed or chair.

aptation to aerobic training.[12] The training effects of aerobic exercise can allow patients with angina pectoris to perform more intense activity in a pain-free range and they may require less drug therapy to lower myocardial oxygen consumption. This is apparent after a conditioning program when patients are able to perform longer on a stress test at a lower RPP than prior to training.

The improved efficiency of the cardiopulmonary-vascular system after an exercise training program can often compensate for impaired left ventricular function caused by an infarction and thereby allow many patients to function at least at a premorbid level of activity and in some sedentary individuals at higher functional levels than achieved prior to their MI when no left ventricular impairment was present.

The New York Heart Association (NYHA) has developed a system that classifies a patient's overall disability according to functional capacity and therapeutic class (Table 4.11). Safe participation in an aerobic exercise program may result in a higher therapeutic classification as a result of an improved functional capacity.

## Emotional Benefits

As patients with CAD become more comfortable in performing a variety of activities, their fear of the disease lessens and their confidence in their health increases. Families also learn from observation and participation in exercise activities and are reassured of the patient's improved health.

Patients who continue to have chest pain symptoms with exercise learn their exercise limits. Some may not completely adjust to having angina but, learn to respect what the symptom implies. They are more likely to report and respond to the symptom than to deny its presence. This gives family members further confidence in the patient's judgment and can ease the fears that chest pain precipitates.

## Invasive Monitoring

When chest pain warrants hospitalization for management, hemodynamic monitoring may be indicated. This is done in the intensive care unit and can entail serious risks to the patient, including infection, embolism, and dislodgement of the indwelling catheter.

### Swan-Ganz Catheter

The Swan-Ganz catheter provides direct measurement of the central venous pressure of the right side of the heart and the pulmonary artery and indirect measurement of left atrial pressure by placement of the transducer in a branch of the pulmonary artery (pulmonary capillary wedge pressure). The catheter is typically introduced into a peripheral arm vein. By a series of balloon tip inflations and deflations during advancement through the heart, the changes in graphic pressure recordings indicate the location of the catheter tip in the heart (see Fig. 2.8 and Table 2.1.). Blood samples from the various catheter locations in the heart can be obtained by this method for blood gas analysis. Calculations based on the Fick principle can then be made to determine cardiac output and stroke volume.

When potent medications are used hemodynamic monitoring is essential so that results can be immediately observed and drug dosages adjusted. Use of vasopressor agents such as norepinephrine (Levophed) and isoproterenol (Isuprel), which may have adverse effects on the heart, require invasive monitoring. Patients with severe chest pain requiring large amounts of nitrate and morphine therapy for pain relief may have a marked reduction in preload and require fluid replacement to maintain adequate blood pressure. Direct monitoring of cardiac pressures during fluid administration allow early recognition and prevention of heart failure due to fluid overload.

Mobilization of patients with a Swan-Ganz catheter is limited but possible as long as ventricular function can be measured by indirect monitoring of left atrial pressures.

### Arterial Lines

Direct arterial blood pressure measurements can also be recorded from an indwelling arterial catheter. Accurate BP determinations are essential when using potent vasopressors and fluid therapy in patients with CHF. In addition, an ABG determination is readily obtainable in acutely ill patients by an indwelling arterial catheter. Since arterial puncture can be painful and risky, an arterial line is preferred when repeated blood sampling is required, as in evaluating an acute patient response to oxygen and drug therapy.

# Invasive Procedures

## Intra-aortic Balloon Pump

The intra-aortic balloon pump (IABP) is a device used to reduce the work of the heart in the acute care setting, either in the operating room or intensive care unit. It is reserved primarily for patients in cardiogenic shock from an acute MI, those with intractable angina nonresponsive to medication, and those who are difficult to wean from cardiopulmonary bypass.

The IABP consists of an internal catheter in the thoracic aorta and an externally powered pressure system, which triggers timed inflations and deflations of the long balloon component surrounding the distal end of the catheter.

This counterpulsation device is considered a temporary measure to allow the heart to rest and heal. There is a 10 percent morbidity rate from complications of the IABP.[9] Associated risks of the procedure include dislodgement of the balloon to a more distal position in the aorta, causing renal artery obstruction and renal failure; possible aortic rupture; lower extremity ischemia; dissection of aorta, iliac, or femoral arteries; and thrombosis. Risks of these complications increases each day that the patient requires the IABP support. When an IABP is in place, patients should not flex at the trunk by an angle of more than 45° and must keep full extension in the leg harboring the device.

## Pacemaker

The patient with CAD may need temporary pacemaker assistance during an acute ischemic event, or if the blood supply to conduction tissue is completely obstructed, a permanent pacemaker may be necessary. Pacemakers are battery-operated devices that stimulate conduction tissue to produce a muscular contraction when the heart's natural pacemaker fails. (See Ch 7.)

Pacemaker wires are typically placed in the heart during CABGS (discussed below). Although a temporary pacemaker may not be used postoperatively, epicardial pacemaker wires remain in place for several days after surgery. External wires may be seen on these patients' chests but are not attached to the power source unless pacing becomes necessary. In general, patients may be mobilized in spite of the wires, and the temporary pacemaker does not restrict activity as long as the cardiac status is stable.

## Endocardial Muscle Biopsy

Although not frequently performed, a biopsy of endocardial tissue can be useful in the evaluation of myocarditis when it is the suspected cause of chest pain. In this procedure a catheter is introduced into the heart, and several samples of muscle are taken from the right ventricle. The specimen is reviewed for histologic composition and diagnosis. Patients who receive a heart transplant undergo routine right ventricular biopsy for evaluation of rejection and the efficacy of pharmacologic treatment.

The procedure is usually well tolerated and may be performed on an outpatient basis on some individuals.

## Percutaneous Transluminal Coronary Angioplasty

Percutaneous transluminal coronary angioplasty (PTCA) is a procedure performed in the cardiac catheterization laboratory under direct fluoroscopic observation. It is generally used for the patient with a stable lesion in an effort to increase coronary artery blood flow. On occasion it is used during an acute MI in an attempt to preserve as much myocardium as possible.[13] During the procedure a special balloon catheter is guided to the site of the coronary artery lesion. The balloon is repeatedly inflated at the narrowed portion of the vessel. This forces the "plaque" back into the vessel wall. There is a 10 percent risk to the patient for complications, including coronary artery dissection, MI, or hemorrhage. In some cases emergency CABG may be necessary.[14]

The ideal candidate for the procedure is someone with single-vessel, noncalcified atherosclerotic disease in a proximal artery. As skill and technology improve, the procedure is becoming safer to use with a riskier population, including those with multivessel disease, calcified lesions, and distal disease. There is an 80 percent success rate for reduction in lesion size and improvement in coronary artery blood flow after the first time the procedure is performed. A 90 percent success rate is achieved with these procedures if patients requiring repeat dilation within a short period of time (30 days) are included in the calculations.[15] The PTCA procedure has been successfully used in patients whose bypass grafts have developed atherosclerotic disease.[16]

Without complications, the patient typically is in the hospital for 2 to 3 days and returns home on minimal medication since higher myocardial oxygen demands can be met by the improved coronary blood supply. Usually activity limitations are minimal and convalescence takes approximately 1 week. Antiplatelet therapy is instituted to reduce the likelihood of clot formation at the traumatized coronary artery site.

## Coronary Artery Bypass Graft

The CABG has become a relatively routine procedure in the management of incapacitating angina pectoris. When the surgery is performed with skill in facilities doing a high volume of procedures and in low-risk patients, morbidity rates may be as low as 1 to 3 percent.[9] Relief of angina is provided in 85 percent of cases and mortality is decreased in patients with left main coronary artery disease, or triple vessel disease. The Coronary Artery Surgery Study (CASS) was a multicentered randomized trial undertaken to compare outcomes of patients treated medically or surgically. Patients with left main disease or incapacitating angina were excluded from the study. No statistically significant differences were found between the two groups regarding morbidity or mortality when patients met the following criteria:

1. Single- or double-vessel disease
2. Ejection fraction greater than 40 percent
3. Signs and symptoms of ischemia absent on ETT until the heart rate reached at least 120 beats per minute or a 5-MET workload was completed[17]

A CABG is performed with the patient under general anesthesia and requires cardiopulmonary extracorporeal circulatory assistance while the body temperature is lowered and the heart is asystolic. The heart is exposed via a sternal incision simultaneously with harvesting of the saphenous vein. This vein is sewn into the proximal aorta and anastamosed to the coronary artery distal to its obstruction. When possible, the left internal mammary artery (LIMA) is used to bypass the lesion. It is more desirable to use an artery than a vein graft as a vascular conduit for several reasons: (1) a better tolerance to high pressures and (2) a more appropriate response to autonomic stimulation. In addition, the LIMA is anatomically in close proximity to the heart so that extensive leg incisions are not necessary.[18] Prior to surgical closure, blood flow is measured through the new "arterial" supply to ensure patency. When the procedure is completed, the patient is rewarmed and removed from the bypass pump machine. The heart is defibrillated and the patient is transferred to the intensive care unit on ventilatory, antiarrhythmia, and vasopressor support (Fig. 4.6).

An uncomplicated recovery generally requires 7 days of hospitalization devoted to pulmonary hygiene; gradual mobilization and increased activities of daily living; heart rate, rhythm, and blood pressure stabilization during mobilization; wound management; and patient and family education. Patients should be able to easily distinguish their "new" incisional chest pain from preoperative ischemia-induced chest pain. Table 4.12 lists factors related to postoperative angina.

Cardiac conditions that preclude CABG in the presence of recurrent angina and bypassable anatomy include severely depressed left ventricular function, large left ventricular volume, and cardiac failure due to CAD cardiomyopathy. An alternative procedure to relieve angina in these patients may be PTCA.

### Cardiac Transplantation

Cardiac transplantation has become a treatment alternative for patients with severe left ventricular failure and NYHA functional class IV. Patients accepted as candidates for transplantation are expected to have a limited survival beyond 6 months if they do not have surgery. Postoperative recipient

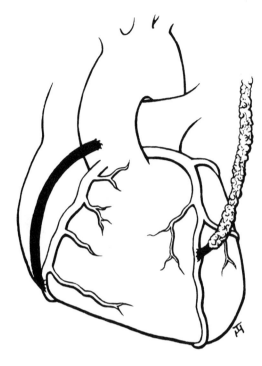

**Fig. 4.6** A saphenous vein graft is shown between the aorta and distal right coronary artery. An internal mammary artery with surrounding soft tissue for protection has been anastomosed to the anterior descending coronary artery. (Reproduced from Collins J: Coronary Bypass Surgery. Physicians East: J Phys Int 5(4-5):6, April–May 1983)

survival rate has been reported as 67 percent in the first year and 54 percent at 5 years.[19]

Early postsurgical management is focused on prevention and treatment of acute rejection of the donor heart and adjustment of immunosuppressive drug regimen. Patients require pulmonary hygiene and general strengthening. The deconditioning that occurred gradually as the patient's heart function deteriorated preoperatively responds well to an endurance exercise program. Postoperative complaints of chest pain are usually due to the sternal incision and musculoskeletal manipulation during surgery. Coronary insufficiency does not present as chest pain owing to cardiac denervation.

Long-term management of these patients includes prevention of donor

**Table 4.12 Factors Relating to Early and Late Postoperative Angina Pectoris**

Resumption of cigarettes
Intraoperative myocardial infarction
Poor distal segment of the coronary artery receiving the anastomosis
Relatively low blood flow in the graft during surgery (<75 ml/min)
Incomplete revascularization of all available arteries during surgery

(Modified from Sokolow M, McIlroy M: Clinical Cardiology. © by Lange Medical Books, Los Altos, CA, 1981.)

heart rejection and prevention of CAD. The latter is the primary cause of late mortality in this population. Since patients lack an "anginal" warning system for myocardial ischemia, periodic exercise tests and/or coronary angiography are used to follow the development and progression of CAD in the transplanted heart.

## PHYSICAL THERAPY INTERVENTION

Physical therapy management of the patient with acute or chronic chest pain can be anxiety-producing if the therapist is unsure of the significance of this symptom. The more information the therapist is able to obtain from the physician, medical records, and patient, the more objective the therapist can be in treating patients with angina pectoris.

## Interview

In addition to the components of the patient interview that are described in Chapter 3, the following key questions can assist the therapist to obtain specific information about this patient's symptoms and should be added to the generic physical therapy patient interview.

1. Where is your chest pain? (Have patient place his own hand on involved areas.)
2. Under what conditions do you get chest pain?
3. What do you do when you experience chest pain?
4. How long does your chest pain last?
5. Is your chest pain frightening to you?
6. What do you think is causing your chest pain?
7. Did you ever injure your chest or have surgery?

## Evaluation

The patient with angina pectoris requires musculoskeletal, cardiopulmonary, and functional evaluations.

### Musculoskeletal Evaluation

In addition to the factors considered in Chapter 3, cervical disc disease and arthritic changes can mimic atypical chest pain of angina pectoris. Range of motion of the neck and shoulders should be performed to help the therapist distinguish symptoms due to coronary ischemia from those of postural malalignment.

## *Cardiopulmonary Evaluation*

### Inspection

The findings of the cardiopulmonary inspection in patients with angina or acute MI are usually normal. When cardiac output is depressed, patients may look pale, ashen, or cyanotic and may be using accessory muscles to breathe. There may be jugular venous distention with right ventricular congestive failure or a displaced cardiac apical pulsation with left ventricular failure or hypertrophy. If chest pain is caused by a pulmonary embolism or a surgical wound, there may be asymmetric thoracic excursion and muscle splinting.

### Palpation

Patients with stable angina usually do not present any findings on palpation unless there are associated findings of prior MI with apical aneurysm or a history of LV hypertrophy. An impulse may be felt at the apex of the heart owing to the discoordinate movement of the aneurysm. With LV hypertrophy, the apex of the heart and the point of maximal impulse (PMI) may be felt closer to the left midaxillary line than to the normal left midclavicular line. During acute myocardial ischemia these findings may become more pronounced.

It is also helpful to apply gentle but firm pressure with the heel of the hand directly over and around the sternum to see if a chest pain symptom can be reproduced. Any localized areas of muscle spasm or tenderness should be palpated to determine other possible causes of angina-like chest pain.

The radial pulse should be evaluated for rate, rhythm, and presence as compared with the apical pulse heard with the stethoscope. Patients with stable angina may reveal no distinguishing findings at peripheral artery palpation. Knowledge of the patient's typical heart rate and rhythm can reassure the therapist of the patient's current stability. During acute coronary insufficiency, the pulse may become rapid, slow, or irregular, and the skin can be damp, clammy, and cold.

### Auscultation

**Heart Sounds.**   Cardiac auscultation should be performed before and after exercise. Patients with stable angina pectoris may reveal no abnormal heart sounds. During an acute episode of coronary insufficiency, an S4 may be heard; the appearance of a new S3 indicates heart failure. Changes in heart sounds, including the onset of an S4, S3, or new murmur should be documented. (see Ch. 2.)

**Lung Sounds.**   There are no alterations in lung sounds in the patient with angina pectoris unless pulmonary edema and/or CHF are associated with the event (see Ch. 5).

Vital Signs

**Blood Pressure.** The patient with stable angina pectoris typically has a normal blood pressure. It may be low depending on the patient's medication. The therapist should be aware of recent blood pressure findings to check for consistency of readings. During acute coronary insufficiency the blood pressure is often elevated. If there is associated heart failure, systolic blood pressure may be low. When anxiety accompanies chest pain, it may cause high blood pressure.

Electrocardiogram

Patients with stable angina pectoris rarely show any abnormalities on a single-lead ECG rhythm strip. During acute chest pain, changes in heart rate (HR) and rhythm consistent with myocardial irritability can be observed. Evaluation of ST segment changes on single-lead telemetry systems is not as reliable as a multilead system in verifying myocardial ischemia, but such changes should be considered during the evaluation.

## Functional Evaluation

The functional evaluation yields important information necessary to develop the physical therapy program. It provides the baseline data regarding the patient's current level of activity and hemodynamic and symptomatic tolerance to the activity. This is useful in establishing safe activity levels as well as in setting limits for long-term endurance training programs.

The hospitalized patient who has been acutely ill and is just beginning to be mobilized may be evaluated daily for tolerance to low-level tasks such as dangling at the bedside, sitting in a chair or bedside commode, taking a few steps, standing at the sink, and performing simple personal hygiene activities. Progressive tasks used to evaluate the patient for tolerance include showering, climbing stairs and ramps, prolonged ambulation, restorator use, and stationary bicycling. When other physical disabilities are present, tolerance to comparable functional activities is monitored. This may include transfers in the case of the amputee or hemiplegic patient, wheelchair propulsion, or ambulation with assistive devices.

Exercises that require isometric contractions or Valsalva maneuvers should be avoided owing to their potent effect on blood pressure. When they must be performed, as in ambulation with crutches, the activity should be monitored.

Before hospital discharge patients may perform a standard low-level exercise test with 12-lead ECG recording and blood pressure measurement. This will provide HR, blood pressure, and RPP guidelines for a safe home exercise program. The type of submaximum test protocol frequently used has the patient work up to a 5-MET work load. A patient who completes the protocol without signs or symptoms of ischemia is allowed to perform

Table 4.13 Effect of Drug Interventions upon Exercise Responses

| Effect | Medication |
|---|---|
| May increase HR | Isoproterenol |
| | Quinidine and procainamide |
| | Bronchodilators and drugs for asthma |
| | Thyroid-synthroid, thyroid USP |
| | Apresoline |
| May decrease HR | Propranolol and other β-blocking agents |
| | Reserpine |
| | Some antihypertensives (e.g., guanethidine, Aldomet) |
| May decrease BP | Aldomet |
| | Apresoline |
| | Propranolol |
| | Diuretics |
| | Nitrates |
| May increase BP | Bronchodilators: epinephrine, aminophylline |
| | Nasal sprays, decongestants, Neo-Synephrine |
| May increase exercise capacity | Nitrates |
| | β-Adrenergic blocking agents |
| | Digitalis: Lanoxin, digitoxin |
| May increase cardiac contractility | Digitalis |
| | Isoproterenol |
| | Aminophylline-type drugs |
| May decrease cardiac contractility | Propranolol and other β-blockers |
| | Procainamide and other antidysrhythmics |

exercise in a monitored program maintaining the HR below that achieved at 5 METs. When a low-level test is positive for ischemia, the patient will most likely have additional evaluative tests, since this presents an increased risk of early morbidity or mortality. However, exercise can safely be performed if the HR intensity is kept to 70 to 85 percent of the maximum safe HR achieved on the low-level ETT. When an ETT is not available, the safe upper limit of an exercise HR may be determined from Holter monitor results or results of a functional evaluation.

A functional evaluation is important in early convalescence in order to determine the work intensity, HR, RPP, and RPE at which the patient shows signs and symptoms of ischemia. The formula for age-predicted maximum exercise HR (220 − age) is inappropriate during this early recovery period and in patients who take drugs affecting the cardiac response to exercise. Table 4.13 lists these drugs and their influence on exercise responses.

Once the safe upper limit has been determined, home activities and an aerobic exercise program can be prescribed. The activity program in the first 1 to 2 months is progressed according to the patient's recovery and the complexity of event.

The intent of an exercise program begun in this early convalescent period is to introduce patients to habitual exercise as well as to achieve initial training effects. This program should include:

1. Exercise using large muscles in a dynamic pattern

**Table 4.14 Characteristics of Below-Knee Amputee Ambulation With and Without Prosthesis**

| Characteristic | With Prosthesis | Without Prosthesis (axillary crutches) | P value |
|---|---|---|---|
| Velocity (m/min)[a] | 71 ±[c] 10 | 71 ± 11 | NS[b] |
| Heart rate (beats/min) | 106 ± 10 | 135 ± 22 | .001 |
| Respiratory rate (breaths/min) | 16 ± 3 | 23 ± 9 | .02 |
| Blood pressure (mmHg) | 146/87 ± 23/11 | 152/86 ± 20/8 | NS |
| Energy cost (ml $O_2$/kg/min) | 15.5 ± 2.8 | 22.3 ± 4.0 | .001 |
| % predicted max $\dot{V}O_2$ | 36 ± 9 | 59 ± 16 | .001 |

[a] Self-selected velocity.
[b] Not significant.
[c] ± standard deviation.
(Adapted from Pagliarulo M, Waters R, Hislop H: Energy cost of walking of below knee amputees having no vascular disease. Phys Ther 59: 538, 1979.)

2. Intensity according to functional evaluation or ETT results in HR, RPP, RPE, or METs (usually less than that required to achieve major cardiovascular benefits)
3. Duration and frequency according to tolerance for activities, usually 1 hour, 5 days per week, at low intensity

After 6 to 8 weeks of convalescence from an acute cardiac event, the myocardium is usually adequately healed for the patient to begin a more intensive aerobic exercise program. A maximum exercise test is typically performed and the training HR range is established at 70 to 85 percent of the maximum HR achieved before signs or symptoms of myocardial ischemia appear. These may include angina associated with 1 mm of horizontal ST segment depression, a drop in blood pressure with increasing work, or exercise-induced dysrhythmias. Since many cardiopulmonary medications can affect the cardiac response to exercise, it is important for patients to take their routine medications for the ETT in order for the exercise training HR to be accurate.

Patients taking β-adrenergic blocking drugs have a lower resting and exercise HR. It has been well documented that patients using these drugs can achieve the benefits of aerobic exercise when they train at 70 to 85 percent of the HR safely achieved on the ETT even though the chronotropic response is blunted.

The intensity of exercise is only one component of the exercise prescription. In order to achieve cardiovascular benefits of an aerobic program, the elevated HR must be maintained for 30 minutes three to five times per week.

A functional evaluation is invaluable even when a standard ETT has been done. It can be used to apply exercise limits determined from the stress test to other modalities. For example, a patient may safely achieve an RPP of 12,000 on an ETT (treadmill). A functional evaluation can then be done to translate 9 minutes of graded treadmill walking to 30 minutes of stationary bicycling, keeping the RPP less than 12,000. Heart rate and (systolic) blood pressure (SBP) responses to the two different modalities may vary when an RPP of 12,000 is achieved.

| Exercise Example | HR (beats/min) | × SBP (mmHg) | = | RPP |
|---|---|---|---|---|
| Exercise tolerance test: low-level treadmill, work load 1.7 mph on 10% grade (peak) | 100 | × 120 | = | 12,000 |
| Functional evaluation: stationary bicycle, work load freewheel at 50 rpm | 80 | × 150 | = | 12,000 |

The above example shows that the patient may need to work at a lower HR when riding the bicycle than when walking. This information is extremely helpful if the patient lives up several flights of stairs, in a hilly neighborhood, or in a very cold climate, where stationary bicycling is more realistic than a walking program. The functional evaluation also tells us that this patient would just need to freewheel to achieve the desired RPP.

A functional evaluation for planning an alternative aerobic exercise program can be performed and may include arm pedaling, leg restorator pedaling, wheelchair propulsion, swimming, use of a cross-country skiing simulator, work with arm pulleys, or ambulation with assistive devices. It should be kept in mind that various physical disabilities may impose higher energy demands for performing similar tasks. Table 4.14 illustrates this in below-knee amputee ambulation with or without a prosthesis. Patients with physical disabilities require more energy to perform functional tasks. They should be allowed to choose their most comfortable pace for the activity, as this will be the most energy-efficient pace.[20,21] Numerous parameters are monitored during the functional evaluation. The evaluation should be performed at least 1 hour after a meal and with all usual medicines. Table 4.15 lists these parameters.

The functional evaluation is terminated when symptoms or signs of intolerance appear. These may include fatigue, breathlessness, irregular heart beat, chest pain, lightheadedness, or leg pain. It is important to remember that any patient may deny symptoms, which necessitates close observation of objective measurements.

Patients can be given an independent exercise program to do daily to

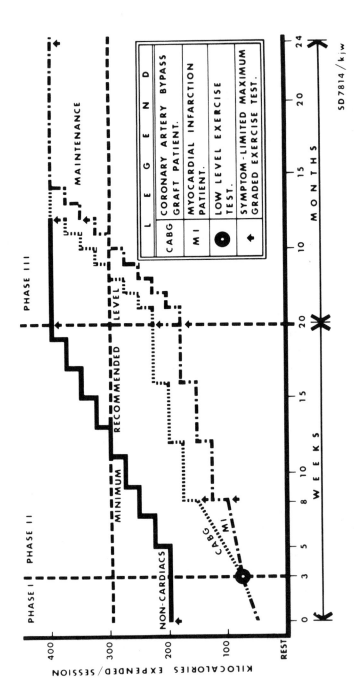

**Fig. 4.7** Progression in aerobic training in noncardiac and cardiac patients. (Reproduced from Pollock M, Ward A, Foster C: Exercise prescription for rehabilitation of the cardiac patient. In Pollock M, Schmidt D (eds): Heart Disease and Rehabilitation. Houghton-Mifflin, Boston, 1979)

**Table 4.15 Parameters Monitored during Functional Evaluation**

| | |
|---|---|
| Heart rate | Heart rhythm |
| Blood pressure | Respiratory rate |
| Heart sounds | Breath sounds |
| Color | Coordination |
| Orientation | Skin temperature |
| Symptoms of | |
|     Chest pain | Breathlessness |
|     Local muscle pain | Fatigue |
|     Diaphoresis | Lightheadedness |

complement activities performed in therapy. Patients are instructed in self-monitoring techniques for heart rate, rhythm, RPE scale, and symptom recognition and are given limits for each of these parameters to ensure a safe program. In cases in which angina symptoms severely restrict activity performance, prophylactic nitroglycerin may be useful. Figure 4.7 illustrates the progression in aerobic training in cardiac and noncardiac patients. Phases 1, 2, and 3 in the figure reflect the recovery process from a cardiac event, including the acute, convalescent, and conditioning phases and maintenance periods. The physical therapist is integrally involved in all phases of the total conditioning process.

# REFERENCES

1. Ganong W: Review of Medical Physiology. 8th Ed. Lange Medical Books, Los Altos, CA. 1977
2. Breidenbaugh P: Musculoskeletal Chest Pain in Patients with Visceral Sources Ruled Out. Thesis, Medical College of Virginia, Richmond, 1984
3. Hart F (ed): French's Index of Differential Diagnosis. 10th Ed. John Wright & Sons, Bristol, 1973
4. Ellestad M: Stress Testing. Principles and Practice. 2nd Ed. FA Davis, Philadelphia, 1980
5. Theroux P, Waters D, Halphen C, et al: Prognostic valve of exercise testing soon after MI. N Engl J Med 301:341, 1979
6. American College of Sports Medicine: Guidelines for Graded Exercise Testing and Exercise Prescription. Ed. Lea & Febiger, Philadelphia
7. Wisenberg G, Schelbert H, Radionuclide Techniques in the Diagnosis of Cardiovascular Disease. Curr Prob Cardiol 4:(7)25 1979
8. Pandian, N: Diagnostic role of color Doppler echocardiography. (Abstr.) In New England Cardiovascular Society, Symp On Recent Advances in Cardiovascular Disease—1987. American Heart Association, Massachusetts Affiliate, 1987
9. Sokolow M, McIlroy M: Clinical Cardiology. Lange Medical Books, Los Altos, CA, 1981

10. Rehabilitation of Patients with Cardiovascular Disease. Reports of a WHO Committee. World Health Organization Technical Report Series #278, Geneva, 1974
11. Paffenbarger R, Hyde R, Wing A, et al: Physical activity, all-cause mortality, and longevity of college alumini. N Engl J Med 314:605, 1986
12. Hagberg J, Ehsani A, Holloszy J: Effects of 12 months of intense exercise training on stroke volume in patients with CAD. Circulation 67:1194, 1983
13. Topol E, Califf R, George B, et al, A randomized trial of immediate vs. delayed elective angioplasty after IV TPA in acute MI. N Engl J Med 317:581, 1987
14. Rapaport E: Percutaneous Transluminal Coronary Angioplasty. Circulation 60(5), 1979, p 969
15. Berger E, Williams D, Reinert S, et al: Sustained efficacy of percutaneous transluminal coronary angioplasty. Am Heart J 111:233, 1986
16. Williams D: Current status of PTCA, (Abstr.) New England Cardiovascular Society, Scientific Session. In Recent Advances in Cardiovascular Diseases—1987 American Heart Association, Massachusetts Affiliate, 1987
17. CASS principal Investigators and Associates: Coronary Artery Surgery Study (CASS): a Randomized Trial of CABS. Survival Data. Circ 68 (5):939–950, 1983
18. Collins J: Coronary Bypass Surgery. Physicians East: J Phys Int 5 (4–5):6 1983
19. Baumgartner W, Reitz B, Oyer P, et al. Cardiac homotransplantation. Surgery 16(9):6, 1979
20. Fisher S, Gullickson G: Energy cost of ambulation in health and disability. A literature review. Arch Phys Med Rehabil 59: March 1978
21. Energy Cost: Studies Related to Physical Therapy An Anthology. American Physical Therapy Association Alexandria, VA, 1981

## SUGGESTED READINGS

Amsterdam E, Wilmont J, DeMaria A: Exercise in Cardiovascular Health and Disease, Yorke Medical Books, New York, 1977
Amundsen L (ed): Cardiac Rehabilitation. Churchill Livingstone, New York, 1981
Cardiac Rehabilitation Phys Ther J Monogr: American Physical Therapy Association, Alexandria, VA, Dec. 1985
Irwin S, Tecklin J: Cardiopulmonary Physical Therapy. CV Mosby, St. Louis, 1985
Pollock M, Schmidt D (eds): Heart Disease and Rehabilitation. Houghton-Mifflin Boston, 1979
Vinsant M, Spence M, Hagen D: A Common Sense Approach to Coronary Care. A Program. 2nd Ed., CV Mosby, St. Louis, 1975
Wenger N (ed): Exercise and the heart. Cardiovasc Clin: FA Davis, Philadelphia, 1985

# BREATHLESSNESS 5

Breathlessness is often referred to either as shortness of breath (SOB) or as dyspnea. For any of us who engage in fairly strenuous exercise it is a common experience, yet it can be a terribly frightening experience, and one that patients avoid if at all posssible. It is accompanied by the fear of suffocation and all the discomforts of that fear. A large number of conditions, some quite benign but others indicative of a serious problem, can result in breathlessness. Table 5.1 below describes the differential diagnosis.

## CHART REVIEW

Breathlessness can be a very acute problem, in choking victims, leaving little time to properly perform patient examinations. However, previous knowledge from a patient's chart regarding his history, cardiopulmonary status, and the results of various tests can quickly direct the physical therapist to a correct analysis of the cause of the patient's dyspnea, and to an appropriate solution.

### Medical History

Important to the etiology of breathlessness or cough is whether or not the patient smokes or ever smoked and if so, what, how much, and for how long. Cigarettes are more damaging to lungs than cigars or pipes, largely because of the way in which inhalation is habitually done. In a medical history, the unit of smoking over time is often the pack-year, which is the number of years times the number of packs of cigarettes smoked per day. Thus, if a patient smoked two packs daily for 40 years, he has a $2 \times 40 = 80$ pack-year history. The higher the pack-year exposure, the more damage to tissue is likely, although there is probably a genetic predisposition to some lung diseases.

Exposure to environmental substances can be significant in breathlessness and should be noted in the medical history. Asbestos exposure produces significant deterioration of lung tissue, resulting in loss of gas-exchanging

**Table 5.1 Differential Diagnosis of Breathlessness**

| Possible Causes | Possible Findings | Stimuli | Pathology |
|---|---|---|---|
| Increased metabolic demand for oxygen | Increased respiratory rate; increased heart rate; increased blood pressure; use of accessory muscles; possible paradoxical abdominal motion | Exercise<br>Fever | Normal<br>Infection<br>Hypoxia |
| Left ventricular dysfunction | Ventricular dilatation; symmetrical rales; S3, S4 gallop; fatigue; decreased blood pressure; increased heart rate; increased respiratory rate; poor diaphragm excursion | Chronic hypertension<br>Exercise<br>Chronic fluid retention | Left ventricular congestive heart failure<br>Valve stenosis<br>Valve incompetence |
| Bronchospasm | Inspiratory/expiratory wheeze; tight cough; mucoid, sparse, or copious sputum | Exercise<br>Airborne irritants<br>Forced expiration<br>Bronchial irritation<br>Drugs (β blockers) | Asthma<br>Allergic reaction |
| Hyperventilation | Increased respiratory rate disproportionate to level of exertion; pallor; diaphoresis; lightheadedness; may have loss of consciousness | Anxiety<br>Fever<br>Hypercapnia<br>Hypoxia | Restrictive lung disease<br>Metabolic or respiratory acidosis |
| Choking | No verbalization; ineffective breathing effort; nasal flares; rib retractions | Foreign object or tongue in airway | None |
| Inadequate gas exchange in lung | Resting breathlessness; $PO_2 < 55$ mmHg; accessory muscle use; increased HR; cyanosis; drowsiness; confused or unconscious; chest x-ray abnormality | Lung disease<br>Cardiac arrest<br>Anesthesia<br>Hypoxia<br>Fatigue of muscles of ventilation | Respiratory failure<br>COPD<br>Pneumonia<br>Asbestosis |
| Lung collapse from loss of pressure gradient | Decreased movement on one side of chest; rapid onset; no pain; no cough; decreased breath sounds; increased percussion resonance | Spontaneous chest trauma<br>Pre-existing lung disease (cystic fibrosis) | Pneumothorax |
| Obstruction in pulmonary circulation with interruption of blood flow | Sudden onset of breathlessness; chest pain; cough; hemoptysis; fever; loss of consciousness; increased HR; V/Q shows increased dead space; angiography shows lesion | Prolonged bedrest<br>Recent MI<br>Chronic CHF<br>Atrial fibrillation<br>Fracture of long bone<br>Recent surgery | Pulmonary embolus |

function. Hypoxia and the need for supplemental oxygen is common in this group of patients. In addition, there are "black lung" of the coal miner, "white lung" of the baker, "farmer's lung" in tobacco farming, and perhaps more obscure causes of lung diseases that can be primary causes of breathlessness.

The presence of a cough should be noted. If it is chronic, a description of its features, and any sputum can be very informative (Table 10.1). If it is a new onset, there may be a need for additional diagnostic tests to evaluate its cause including chest x-ray, pulmonary function tests (PFTs), and sputum culture.

## Dyspnea on Exertion (DOE)

The complaint of not being able to breathe enough, of having to breathe too much, or of an abnormal uncomfortable feeling during breathing with exercise is common in patients who have cardiopulmonary dysfunction. The more severe the dysfunction, the less the degree of exertion required to stimulate the complaint. When dyspnea occurs at rest, the compromise to the cardiovascular and/or pulmonary function is most severe. Common experiences among patients include breathlessness with lifting "heavy" objects (isometric contractions with breath holding and Valsalva); breathlessness with stair climbing, becoming severe even if only one or two steps; and breathlessness while walking short distances such as one or two blocks.[1]

An important clue to determining whether the heart or the lungs are contributing most to the symptom is the method the patient uses to obtain relief. If specific breathing patterns are used, such as pursed-lips breathing, and/or if the specific body position of leaning forward on arms to lock the shoulder girdle is used, breathlessness is most likely ventilatory in origin. If cough accompanies the breathlessness, it is helpful to evaluate breath sounds and sputum appearance to differentiate the source (see section on Auscultation in this chapter and Chapter 10).

## Paroxysmal Nocturnal Dyspnea

Breathlessness which awakens the patient after a long period of supine sleep (usually nocturnal) is referred to as *paroxysmal nocturnal dyspnea* (PND). Its frequent occurrence implies congestive heart failure (CHF), in which pulmonary edema is worsened in recumbency owing to hydrostatic shifts in blood volume.

## Orthopnea

Breathlessness that occurs when the patient lies supine and is relieved with one or more pillows propping up the head is referred to as *orthopnea*. Medical histories will refer to "two- or three-pillow" orthopnea as an index of severity. It is similar to PND but is not restricted to nocturnal incidence.

## Implications for Physical Therapy

If the patient's history includes episodes of breathlessness, the therapist may check for the following prior to initiating treatment:

1. What do the PFTs show? Does the patient have chronic obstructive pulmonary disease (COPD)? Or restrictive lung disease? Does the patient show any response to bronchodilator therapy? If there is COPD without bronchodilator response, a complete cardiopulmonary evaluation is indicated to determine whether specific breathing exercises and pulmonary hygiene are needed. If there is a bronchodilator response, the patient may need to use a bronchodilator inhaler prior to performing exercise (see Case 5). Humidity and other environmental conditions as well as hydrotherapy, may cause additional stress.
2. The chest x-ray report should provide information on whether the person has an organic cause for breathlessness. A bronchoscopy could provide a lung biopsy specimen and information on organic disease.
3. The patient's heart rate, blood pressure, and respiratory rate should be checked. If all are elevated, anxiety may be a cause of hyperventilation, especially if diaphoresis and lightheadedness occur.

# Physical Examination

## Patient Appearance

Some, but by no means all, patients who experience breathlessness have clear signs of hypoxemia. Fingernail and toenail clubbing is one sign indicating a chronic state of tissue hypoxemia, and is seen in patients who have a significant degree of shunt in lungs or heart, so that deoxygenated blood is circulated to peripheral tissues. Patients with ventricular septal defects (VSD), cystic fibrosis, severe bronchiectasis, and pulmonary embolism often show this sign. If a reversal of the shunt is possible, as with surgical repair of a VSD, the clubbing disappears.

Patients with COPD may have a primary emphysematous problem and show the "pink puffer" appearance (see Case 2) or may have a high degree of chronic bronchitis with right ventricular dysfunction and show the "blue bloater" appearance (see Ch. 1).

Spinal deformities such as severe kyphoscoliosis can produce such a compromise to ventilation that breathlessness occurs. Obesity likewise can restrict diaphragmatic function and result in unusual degrees of breathlessness.

Combinations of these problems are actually quite common. The patient who is overweight may have CHF accompanied by peripheral edema, clubbing, and cyanosis and may be breathless owing to chronic bronchitis, right ventricular CHF, and obesity.

### Vital Signs

#### Heart Rate

The heart rate can be rapid due to a high state of anxiety that the breathless patient is experiencing, especially when in a panic about not getting enough air. The heart rate may be fast in the breathless patients owing to medications used to produce bronchodilation (see pharmacology in this chapter). Is the heart rate indicative of tachycardia or of normal sinus rhythm and rate? Fever, CHF, and certain medications may produce both breathlessness and tachycardia.

#### Heart Rhythm

Pulmonary patients can have normal sinus rhythm but often show supra-ventricular dysrhythmias due to atrial strain when the pulmonary circulation is involved in the pulmonary pathology (see Ch. 7).

#### Blood Pressure

Is the blood pressure in a normal range for the patient's age? If blood pressure is low, this in combination with breathlessness and other findings can indicate heart failure.

#### Respiratory Rate

Respiratory rate is rapid with breathlessness.

#### Temperature

Is the core temperature normal? An elevation from any origin can cause breathlessness because of increased metabolism, and a primary infection or inflammatory reaction in the lung can produce both breathlessness and fever.

### Auscultation

#### Heart Sounds

There may be documentation of an S3 or S4 or both (gallop rhythm) (see Ch. 4) with breathlessness when this symptom is due to CHF.

#### Breath Sounds

All adventitious breath sounds can be present in isolation or in combination wth breathlessness.

**Normal Breath Sounds.** Vesicular breath sounds are normal inspiratory sounds of air moving within normal small airways and lung parenchyma. Usually little or no sound is heard during most of expiration.

Bronchial breath sounds are similar to the sound that air makes as it travels through the largest airways, especially the trachea. When these sounds are heard anywhere over the thorax, it usually means that lung tissue is consolidated (as in atelectasis), and tubular sounds are transmitted through consolidated tissue.

**Adventitious Breath Sounds.** *Rales* are small-airway abnormal sounds made when fluid is contained within terminal bronchioles and alveoli and resemble the sound of hairs being rubbed together or of cellophane crinkling. Fluid-filled air sacs may indicate pulmonary edema, CHF, or pneumonia, and the sounds they generate are usually heard during inspiration.

*Rhonchi* are rumbling sounds produced when airways contain fluid or mucus secretions. These sounds are often more pronounced during expiration.

*Wheezes* are the musical noises produced by high air flow velocity through constricted airways and can be heard on inspiration and expiration. Wheezes do not necessarily suggest bronchospasm, since retained secretions in airways may also produce wheezing.

## Tests

Medical tests that help to determine whether breathlessness is pulmonary or cardiac or both in origin include (1) arterial blood gases (ABGs); (2) PFTs; and (3) electrocardiograms (ECGs).

### Laboratory Values

### Arterial Blood Gases

Arterial blood gas values are most useful if obtained both resting on room air and during an exercise test because they may be quite normal at rest but show desaturation of oxyhemoglobin with some level of exercise demand for oxygen. The partial pressure of oxygen ($PO_2$) value should always be read with the oxygen dissociation curve as a reference (see Fig. 1.2). The two anchor points on the curve are the point for arterial blood ($PO_2$ 100, $O_2$ saturation 97 percent) and the point for venous blood ($PO_2$ 40, $O_2$ saturation 75 percent). Any $PO_2$ above 60 mmHg means that $O_2$ saturation is probably adequate because the curve is fairly flat, and cyanosis is unlikely to be seen. However $O_2$ saturation may vary and be inadequate when the curve has shifted to the right, which occurs under certain metabolic conditions. The normal value of arterial carbon dioxide pressure ($PCO_2$) is 40 mmHg, with a small range of 37 to 43 unaffected by age. A rise in this value indicates $CO_2$ retention, which can be caused by two major factors, hypoventilation and ventilation/perfusion ($\dot{V}/\dot{Q}$) inequality.

It is possible to have a low $PO_2$ and a high $PCO_2$ from hypoventilation in a patient, but it is only the $PCO_2$ that affects the arterial pH.

Arterial pH

Arterial pH is a measure of the acid-base status of the blood, which is closely linked to the arterial $PCO_2$. For example, respiratory acidosis is caused by $CO_2$ retention, which is brought on by inadequate ventilation when there is a need to blow off more $CO_2$ but that need is not met. As the $PCO_2$ rises, the pH falls (according to the Henderson-Hasselbach equation), so that a doubling of the $PCO_2$ from 40 to 80 mmHg will reduce the pH from 7.4 to about 7.2. This drop is rapidly reversible by hyperventilation. If hyperventilation is impossible owing to disease or muscle weakness or if it simply is not effective owing to $\dot{V}/\dot{Q}$ inequalities, then chronic $CO_2$ retention arises and metabolic compensation eventually takes place through the kidney mechanism of retaining bicarbonate in response to the increase in $PCO_2$ to buffer the acidosis of the blood. The pH is then brought back into line and is kept close to the normal 7.4.

It is also possible to develop a metabolic, not a respiratory, acidosis, as can occur in uncontrolled diabetes mellitus or in anaerobic metabolism with lactic acid production. The drop in pH stimulates the peripheral chemoreceptors to increase the ventilation and lower the $PCO_2$ even if there is no $CO_2$ retention. This could result in tissue hypoxia but usually causes dizziness and loss of consciousness due to blowing off too much $CO_2$. When the ventilatory response is inadequate, the pH does not return to normal, which triggers the need for the metabolic compensation, with kidney retention of bicarbonate.

When arterial pH rises, alkalosis occurs. This could be respiratory, as in hyperventilation, or metabolic, as can occur with severe vomiting. Overventilation of patients on mechanical ventilation or during cardiopulmonary resuscitation (CPR) may result in alkalosis.

Implications for Physical Therapy

Arterial blood gases yield essential information about the patient's adequacy of breathing, and the ability of his lungs to diffuse gases. His need for supplemental oxygen for support of exercise may be clear.

## Pulmonary Function Tests

The standard PFTs (see Ch. 1) may report a flow-volume loop or a normal spirogram tracing of forced vital capacity (FVC). The flow-volume loop indicates FVC and 1-second forced expiratory volume ($FEV_1$) both of which are useful. The patient who has a smaller than predicted FVC has some degree of restrictive lung disease and simply has lost or has never had the predicted lung volume for age, sex, and body height. The patient who has a smaller than predicted $FEV_1$ has obstructive lung disease and has lost the ability to move air through the airways in the lungs (Fig. 5.1). There are many etiologies of obstructive lung disease. Probably most common is a

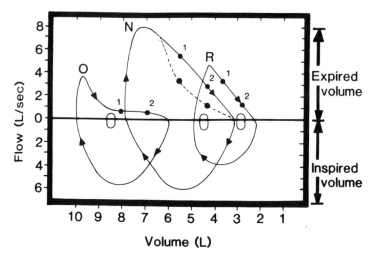

**Fig. 5.1** Flow volume loops normally (N) and in obstructed (O) or restricted (R) pathology. The dashed line on the normal flow-volume curve represents a change that may indicate small airway disease. (Reproduced from Protas EJ: Pulmonary function testing, p. 235. In: Rothstein JM (ed): Measurement in Physical Therapy. Churchill Livingstone, New York, 1985.)

combination of chronic bronchitis and emphysema from a long history of smoking. In addition to the above-mentioned test values, the single-breath diffusion capacity (DLCO) may have been obtained. When this appears lower than predicted, the membrane exchange of $O_2$ and $CO_2$ is impaired.

### Electrocardiograms

Irregular heart beats, such as occurs in paroxysmal atrial tachycardia, and supraventricular tachycardias can be accompanied by breathlessness and are commonly seen in patients with COPD (see Ch. 7).

### V̇O₂ Stress Testing

Impairment of gas exchange may be the cause of breathlessness. To distinguish between a variety of clinical causes, a graded, standardized exercise stimulus in a laboratory that permits the measurement of exercise ventilatory responses and cardiac and pulmonary blood flow responses may be used (see section on Tests).

### Exercise Physiology

Exercise increases the gas exchange requirements in working muscle tissue to provide the energy for performance of the exercise. Oxidative metabolism is the most efficient way to provide energy, although energy is made available in the absence of $O_2$ as well. Since $O_2$ is not stored in any significant quantity in body tissues, it must be delivered via muscle blood flow almost immediately when exercise begins and continuously as exercise goes on.

Muscle blood flow is increased at the start of exercise through vasodilation. The volume of blood moving from the heart to active muscle is also increased by increasing the cardiac output and by redistribution of blood away from viscera and inactive tissue to active muscle, to heart, and to lungs.

The cardiac output increases as the heart rate and stroke volume increase. Stroke volume rises to a maximal plateau soon after exercise begins because venous return is immediately elevated through the active muscle and thoracic pumps. Further increases in cardiac output occur by increasing the heart rate as the oxygen requirement is increased. There is a linear relationship between heart rate and oxygen uptake ($\dot{V}O_2$) up to the maximal values for each individual.

With exercise, right ventricular stroke volume is higher than at rest, and the pulmonary circulation dilates causing recruitment of underperfused lung units. Pulmonary circulation dilation is a normal exercise response which leads to elevation in left ventricular stroke volume.

As pulmonary blood flow increases, ventilation to all lung units proportionally increases. Gas exchange between the pulmonary capillaries and the alveoli is permitted to the exact degree needed to reoxygenate the blood and to eliminate the excess $CO_2$ generated during oxidative metabolism in the working muscle. The elevation in ventilation occurs by an increase in tidal volume at low and moderate exercise intensities and by an increase in respiratory rate at high exercise intensities.

The cardiopulmonary adaptation that occurs at the beginning of exercise persists as the oxygen requirement approaches a steady state. The exactness with which this adaptation is coupled to cellular metabolism makes blood pH, $PCO_2$, and $PO_2$ very stable through low and moderate exercise levels. Only during heavy work (beyond 50 to 60 percent of maximal effort) is a metabolic acidosis seen. At this level of oxygen requirement there is such a high demand for energy that it exceeds the ability of the oxidative metabolic pathway, with its dependence upon the entire oxygen transport system, to meet the demand. Oxygen is delivered but at a rate that lags behind the required rate. To supply the additional energy the anaerobic metabolic pathway is activated as a supplement to the aerobic one. When this recruitment takes place lactate begins to be formed because it is the end product of the anaerobic pathway. The lactate accumulates in muscle and finally in blood, and as it does so, the acid content of blood rises, which shifts the pH to a lower value. The exercise level that shows the rapid rise in blood lactate has been called the *lactate,* or *anaerobic, threshold.*

The effect that lactate accumulation has on breathing is most important. Lactic acid buffering, due to retention of bicarbonate by the kidneys, adds $CO_2$ to the blood in addition to that being produced by aerobic metabolism.

A rise in $CO_2$ produces a ventilatory stimulus to blow off the added $CO_2$ and thus prevent further rise in $PCO_2$ and, in fact, bring it back to its normal value of 40. In addition, the increased hydrogen ion concentration, caused by reduction of blood bicarbonate, stimulates the carotid body mechanism of increasing ventilation to allow for a respiratory compensation for the metabolic acidosis. Therefore, as exercise intensity increases to and above the anaerobic threshold, the ventilation rate starts to increase much more rapidly than the $CO_2$ output, causing $PCO_2$ to decrease. A look at the relationship of the ventilatory stimulus (or degree of metabolic acidosis) to the patient's ventilatory response gives vital information about the source of a complaint of breathlessness. For example, a low degree of stimulus that produces a higher than expected ventilatory response leads to the sensation of breathlessness at relatively low exertional levels.

### Exercise Test Results

During a standard exercise test for evaluation of the causes of dyspnea, a patient pedals a stationary bicycle or walks on a treadmill, beginning at a low intensity of exercise and gradually progressing to maximal intensity, usually with 1-minute increments of increasing work rate (or power). At early low-level exercise patients show the usual submaximal adaptations of the oxygen deficit period, with rise of heart rate, tidal volume, minute ventilation, and oxygen consumption. As the work rate continues to rise, a leveling off to near steady state usually appears, showing an adequate delivery of oxygen and exact coupling of $CO_2$ elimination with cellular energy requirement. Heart rate, minute ventilation, $\dot{V}O_2$ and $\dot{V}CO_2$ rise very gradually and blood lactate remains near initial baseline levels. At anaerobic threshold, lactate begins a rapid accumulation, and minute ventilation rises with a curvilinear adjustment (Fig. 5.2 A, B, C).

The end points for this test are fatigue, dyspnea, or significant cardiac signs or symptoms. To obtain the most complete information for the evaluation of breathlessness, the exercise measures listed in Table 5.2 are taken.

### Interpretation of Exercise Test

**Causes of Dyspnea.** At many points along the oxygen transport system there can be an organic interference with oxygen flow to working muscle. There may also be an organic cause for interference with $CO_2$ elimination. Table 5.3 summarizes the causes and the measurements that deviate from normal.

When heart diseases produce dyspnea on exertion, the basic defect is the problem of a limited cardiac output during exercise, primarily from the reduction in stroke volume. To compensate for a lower stroke volume (SV), a faster than expected heart rate (HR), and a wider than expected arteriovenous $O_2$ difference $[C(a - \bar{v})O_2]$ develop at an inappropriately low work rate.

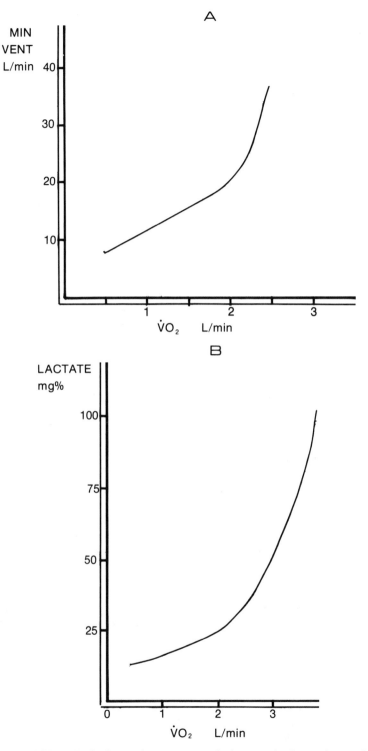

**Fig. 5.2** (**A–E**) Hypothetical exercise responses during standard exercise testing for dyspnea evaluation. A, B show a change from linearity to curvilinearity that identifies the onset of dyspnea. (*Figure continues.*)

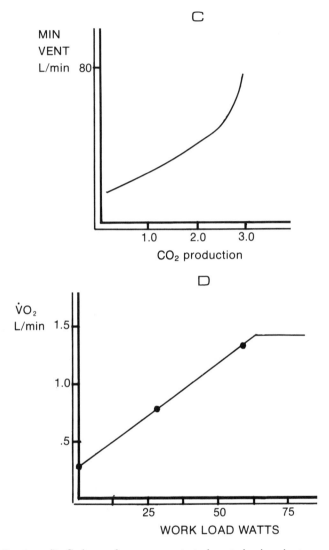

**Fig. 5-2** (*Continued*). C shows dyspnea onset at abrupt rise in minute ventilation. D shows the constant linear relationship between workload and $\dot{V}O_2$ until maximal $\dot{V}O_2$ is reached. (*Figure continues*.)

Working muscle, including muscles of ventilation and myocardium, have difficulty getting an adequate oxygen supply to perform the required work, the anaerobic threshold appears earlier, and dyspnea, fatigue, and even pain may arise. A low anaerobic threshold is common in patients with heart disease or lung disease and in severely deconditioned people. To sort these out, abnormal ECG and blood pressure findings will be most often

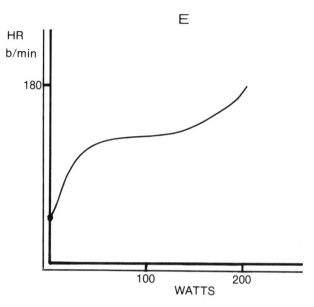

**Fig. 5-2** (*Continued*). E shows how the HR levels off for a brief period of steady state.

found in heart-diseased patients, poor PFT results will be most often found in lung-diseased patients, and fairly normal ECG and PFTs will often occur in deconditioned but otherwise healthy people.

During the incremental stress test, the $\dot{V}O_2$ rises in a linear, predictable pattern, directly proportional to the work rate (see Fig. 5-2 D). If the $\dot{V}O_2$ fails to rise, as work progresses, this may be indicative of cardiac or pe-

**Table 5.2 Exercise Test Measurement Variable**

| **Variable** unit | **Variable** unit |
|---|---|
| Time, minutes | $PO_2$, mmHg |
| Work load, W | $O_2$ saturation, % |
| $O_2$ uptake, ml/min | $PCO_2$, mmHg |
| $CO_2$ output, ml/min | pH |
| Respiratory quotient | $V_D/V_T$, calculated |
| $O_2$ uptake, ml/kg/min | $(A - a)O_2$ gradient, calculated |
| Minute ventilation, L/min | $(A - a)CO_2$ gradient, calculated |
| Respiratory rate, beats/min | $\dfrac{\text{Max min vent}}{\text{MVV}}$, calculated |
| Tidal volume, ml | |
| Heart rate, beats/min | Blood pressure, mmHg |

The endpoint for this test is fatigue, dyspnea, or significant cardiac signs/symptoms. To obtain the most complete information for the evaluation of breathlessness the exercise measures mentioned above are taken. $V_D$ = Dead space ventilation, $V_T$ = Tidal volume, $(A - a)O_2$ gradient = alveolar-arterial $O_2$ gradient, $(A - a)CO_2$ gradient = alveolar-arterial $CO_2$ gradient, Max min vent = maximal minute ventilation.

**Table 5.3 Causes of Dyspnea**

| Disorders | Pathophysiology | Measurements (Deviating from Normal) |
|---|---|---|
| Pulmonary<br>  Air flow limitation | Ventilatory mechanics limit airflow<br>$\dot{V}/\dot{Q}$ mismatch<br>Hypoxia stimulus to breathing | $\dot{V}_E$ max<br>MVV<br>Flow-volume loop in peak exercise<br>$V_D/V_T$<br>$\dot{V}O_2$ max<br>$(A - a)\ O_2$ gradient<br>$\dot{V}_E/\dot{V}O_2$ |
|   Restrictive limitation | $\dot{V}/\dot{Q}$ mismatch | Increased RR<br>$V_D/V_T$ |
| Chest wall<br>  Pulmonary circulation | Mechanical limitation to ventilation | $\dot{V}_E$ max<br>MVV<br>$PaCO_2$<br>$\dot{V}O_2$ max |
| | Rise in physiologic dead space<br>Exercise hypoxemia | $V_D/V_T$<br>$\dot{V}_E/\dot{V}O_2$<br>$PaO_2$ low<br>$O_2$ sat low |
| Cardiac<br>  Coronary | Coronary insufficiency | ECG<br>$\dot{V}O_2$ max<br>Anaerobic threshold<br>$\dot{V}_E/\dot{V}O_2$<br>BP<br>HR |
|   Valvular | $\dot{Q}$ limitation | BP<br>HR |
|   Myocardial | $\dot{Q}$ limitation (decreased ejection fraction) | BP<br>HR |
| Anemia | Decreased $O_2$-carrying capacity | Anaerobic threshold low<br>$\dot{V}O_2$ max<br>$\dot{V}_E/\dot{V}O_2$ |
| Peripheral Circulation | Inadequate blood flow to muscle | $\dot{V}O_2$ max<br>Anaerobic threshold low |
| Obesity | Respiratory restriction<br>Ventiltory insufficiency | $PaO_2$<br>$PaCO_2$<br>$\dot{V}O_2$ max<br>$\dot{V}O_2$ vs. Watts relationship |
| Psychogenic | Hyperventilation | RR<br>$PCO_2$ |
| Malingering | Hyperventilation and hypoventilation<br>Irregular RR | RR<br>$PCO_2$ |
| Deconditioning | Sedentary or bedrest<br>Loss of efficiency of oxygen transport system | Anaerobic threshold low<br>$\dot{V}O_2$ max low |

ripheral vascular limitations. In deconditioned or pulmonary patients, the $\dot{V}O_2$ will be limited to a low maximum but will rise linearly to this point. Limitations may be defined as fatigue (see chapter 6) or due to inadequate gas exchange, poor ventilatory mechanics, or poor peripheral oxygen utilization. Therefore, a low-work-rate anaerobic threshold and a flat $\dot{V}O_2$ below the predicted maximum $\dot{V}O_2$ during the exercise test are specific cardiovascular, not pulmonary, limitations.

The most common reason for dyspnea on exertion in lung or chest wall disorders is mechanical limitation, preventing external respiration from coupling with cellular respiration. Dyspnea is nearly always the primary reason for stopping the exercise test in the pulmonary patient. This symptom appears when the patient cannot eliminate $CO_2$ generated by metabolism. There must be an imbalance between how much breathing must be carried on to eliminate the $CO_2$ being produced by metabolism and how much can be breathed, given the air flow obstruction problem of the patient.

The maximal voluntary ventilation (MVV) is a measure of the patient's maximal breathing capacity at rest, and some patients need to use their total MVV at low levels of exertion. Their minute ventilation ($\dot{V}E$) at maximal effort would then equal their MVV, and there would be no pulmonary reserve. People with no lung disease have a reserve of about 40 percent of their MVV, which means that even at maximal $\dot{V}E$ generated at their maximum $\dot{V}O_2$ they do not nearly approach their MVV and use up just over half of their breathing capacity. The $\dot{V}E$ max/MVV ratio is often called a *dyspnea index* and is generated by a pre-exercise MVV measured with a spirometer (see Ch. 1) and a maximum effort $\dot{V}E$ measured on the continuous incremental exercise test. This index reflects the decreased ventilatory reserve typical of COPD patients.

An increased ventilatory requirement can also lead to dyspnea in which the primary problem is the $\dot{V}/\dot{Q}$ mismatch. When this is present, some regions of the lungs are hypoventilated, while others may be hyperventilated. Simultaneously, the underventilated units cause arterial hypoxemia; this stimulates the carotid body reflex to increase ventilation, which will be greater but ineffectual in diseased lung tissue. For example, the patient with breathlessness on exertion may have the stimulus to ventilate and a responsive respiratory center but an inability to provide an adequate ventilatory response due to mechanical limitations.

When pulmonary patients perform isometric contractions and/or breath-holding maneuvers, commonly during lifting of heavy objects, during sprinting (running to answer the phone), and even during arms-overhead activities, there is no oxidative metabolism supporting the energy requirements of their activity. Since these are examples of anaerobic activities, breathlessness is rapidly brought on by lactate accumulation, the $CO_2$-actuated drive to breathe, and hydrogen ion buffering, with the need for respiratory compensation of a metabolic acidosis. These effects produce potent stimuli to elevate the level of ventilation but pulmonary patients are mechanically unable to breath enough to overcome these metabolic inequalities. Patients simply stop performance, assume postures and patterns of ventilation to support their efforts to restore homeostasis, and take the time necessary to reduce the demands for elevated ventilation.[2,3]

Some patients, owing to spasticity or to loss of a limb, may ride a bicycle ergometer or walk on a treadmill with a great deal of mechanical inefficiency, thus increasing the energy cost of the test beyond expected demand and increasing the likelihood of significant breathlessness earlier than expected in the test.

### Ventilation/Perfusion Scan

A $\dot{V}/\dot{Q}$ scan may have been made. This involves having the patient breathe in a radioactive tracer gas, such as nitrogen 13, and then tracing its distribution in the lung with collimeters, or counters, of radioactivity. Counters are located on both sides of midline, and at specific centimeter intervals from apex to base. Their readings provide a graphic picture of distribution of air, which for upright sitting or standing is not uniform but shows greater ventilation at the apex than at the base. Normally, there is more adequate filling of the base early in a given breath, which would be found using this technique. If there are lung areas receiving reduced ventilation, as in cases of emphysema bullae or tumor, or indeed receiving no ventilation, this scan readily identifies the areas and severity of ventilation deficit. Perfusion is likewise measured with radioactive tracer elements, injected via a venous catheter threaded to the right atrium. A perfusion scan shows whether there are areas of significant dead space, while a ventilation scan shows whether there are areas of significant shunt.

Normally, in the upright posture there is a mismatching of the $\dot{V}/\dot{Q}$ ratio due to the influence of gravity on blood flow distribution in the lung. More blood flows in the dependent sections of the lung, yet the apical lobes of the lung tend to be better ventilated owing to the compliance of lung tissue. With maximal inspiration ventilation is distributed more evenly, and blood flow also may be slightly more evenly distributed. During exercise, in which ventilation becomes higher, there is a tendency to equalize the $\dot{V}/\dot{Q}$ mismatch. In the recumbent position the $\dot{V}/\dot{Q}$ ratio is much more nearly equal than in the upright position.

### Implications for Physical Therapy

The extent of shunt and/or dead space helps decide if oxygen saturation should be monitored during exercise.

### Pulmonary Angiography

A cineangiography study reveals the pathway of radiopaque medium injected into the pulmonary artery as it traverses the entire pulmonary arterial tree. It is precise in identifying the location and size of pulmonary emboli, since these will block the passage of the medium.

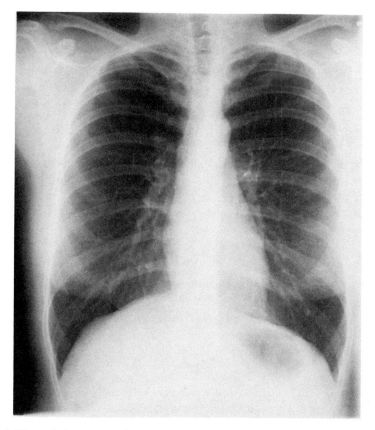

**Fig. 5.3** Normal chest x-ray. Standard anteroposterior film taken in upright position with maximal inspiration.

## Implications for Physical Therapy

Patient may need more oxygen since the embolus may block too much circulation, creating an area of dead space too great to support exercise without supplemental oxygen.

### Chest x-Ray

The chest film should be examined in a systematic way in order to be certain not to miss significant findings. The following structures should be interpreted:

Bony structures and the diaphragm
Heart shadow
Tracheobronchial tree and lung parenchyma (Fig. 5.3)

## Bony Structures

The ribs, clavicles, scapulae, and often the glenohumeral joints are clearly present on most chest films. The vertebral column should be visible through the heart shadow. If a film is overexposed, these bony shadows will be blacked out.

## Diaphragm

Two hemidiaphragms should be well defined by rounded, smooth domes. The right dome is normally situated slightly higher than the left. The costophrenic angle (the junction of the rib cage and the diaphragm) should be clearly delineated.

## Heart Shadow

There should be a sharp definition of cardiac shadow. Standard antero-posterior films will be done in full inspiration and full expiration. A boot-shaped cardiac silhouette signifies left ventricular hypertrophy and may indicate CHF.

## Tracheobronchial Tree

The trachea should be seen as a vertical, translucent shadow in the midline overlying the cervical and upper thoracic vertebrae.

The hili are poorly defined, denser central structures on either side of the midline in the midportion of the central lung field. Each hilum is composed of pulmonary blood vessels, bronchi, and lymph nodes. The tracheal division into right and left main-stem bronchi occurs at the T4 level.

## Lung Parenchyma

Normal lung appears black, with fine white strings fanning out from the hili, which are the *vascular markings*. When these fine, thin markings become fuzzy, they are abnormal.

## Atelectasis

Atelectasis is lung collapse and will appear as a whitened density where black translucence should be. There could be a shift of the mediastinum to the side of the density. More diffuse atelectasis may not be detectable on chest x-ray.

## Infiltrate

Inflammation of lung causes fluid collections in affected areas. This shows up as a density on x-ray but is best differentiated by filling bronchi with air in order to separate consolidated lung tissue from air-filled visible airway tubes. Normally aerated parenchyma will be black, and air-filled bronchi will not be visible but do become visible against a white background of high-density consolidated lung tissue, which cannot be aerated.

## Bullae of Emphysema

Blebs or bullae appear on chest x-ray as nonvascular black, translucent areas, which may be demarcated by a white line.

## Pneumothorax

Introduction of a puncture into the thoracic cavity releases the distending suction that holds lung tissue out against the pleural sheath. Lung collapse results in a mediastinal shift and loss of translucent area where lung tissue should be. The chest film is markedly asymmetric.

## Pleural Effusion

Collections of fluid within the pleural sac occur most often with CHF and are often accompanied by pulmonary edema. This fluid is usually found collecting at the lung bases in upright posture and causes compression and atelectasis of lung tissue. Sometimes fluid may collect locally and be walled off by bridging fibrous tissue. Chest x-ray will show horizontal white lines at fluid borders, called Kerley B lines.[4]

## Implications for Physical Therapy

Findings on chest x-ray help determine whether pulmonary hygiene is necessary

Findings on chest x-ray help decide where pulmonary hygiene will benefit the patient

The presence of the boot-shaped heart and Kerley B lines indicate the need for heart rate, ECG, and blood pressure monitoring during physical therapy procedures.

## *Bronchoscopy*

Fiberoptic bronchoscopy may be used both therapeutically and diagnostically for a variety of purposes. In addition, a rigid bronchoscope may be used for specific situations including foreign body extraction, dilation of a severely stenotic trachea, or biopsy of vascular tumors. The vast majority of bronchoscopy studies are performed with the flexible fiberoptic instrument, which is more versatile, can enter almost three-fourths of fourth-order bronchi, and allows visualization of over half of sixth-order bronchi. The procedure is carried out under local anesthesia, and the flexible bronchoscope is inserted through nostril, mouth, or endotracheal tube to the farthest depth possible. When bronchoscopy is done for diagnostic purposes, sputum or cell samples may be collected from patients with persistent cough, hemoptysis, localized wheezing, or diaphragm paralysis; for airway evaluation during or after intubation; for evaluation of bronchoalveolar lavage; and to obtain selective cultures for infiltrates. Therapeutic indications include patients with excess tenacious secretions, atelectasis, foreign bodies, and bronchoalveolar lavage.

Absolute contraindications for this invasive procedure include: lack of patient cooperation, recent MI (within 6 weeks), significant cardiovascular instability, hypoxemia ($PO_2 < 65$ with supplemental $O_2$), acute hypercapnia ($PCO_2 > 45$), and pulmonary hypertension.

There are risks associated with the procedure, which may preclude the test in certain cases. One risk is that of increased bronchospasm, with a measured drop in pulmonary function. The $FEV_1$ and vital capacity may drop by 30 percent after bronchoscopy. This may lead to cough and dyspnea. There is a 7 percent incidence of postbronchoscopy infiltrate, which may require antibiotic therapy. The majority of patients who undergo bronchoscopy develop sinus tachycardia during and following the procedure. In 1 to 2 percent of the cases, irregular heart beats (supraventricular tachycardia, premature ventricular contractions, and sinus bradycardia) appear.

When bronchoscopy is performed to obtain a biopsy sample, there are additional risks. Complications such as pneumothorax and hemorrhage have been reported. The former has occurred with a 5.5 percent incidence and the latter with a 1.3 percent incidence if significant hemorrhage is defined as greater than 50 to 100 ml of blood. The few deaths reported as a consequence of bronchoscopy have occurred in patients with myocardial disease, severe COPD, serious pneumonia, or cancer.

As technological advances improve the technique, the procedure is being used with less risk for an even greater variety of purposes.[5,6,7]

Implications for Physical Therapy

A common reaction to bronchoscopy is excess airway obstruction, which leads to additional breathlessness and the need for bronchial hygiene and relaxation techniques.

Occasionally, chest physical therapy is performed during bronchoscopy in order to assist the physician to perform the procedure. It may be possible to penetrate to smaller bronchi size with this assistance.

*Sputum Culture*

See Chapter 10.

## MEDICAL-SURGICAL INTERVENTION

# Pharmacology

## Oxygen

Supplemental oxygen is usually indicated for patients who have a resting $PO_2$ of 60 mmHg or less or who desaturate their hemoglobin to 85 percent or less. Patients who have clear diagnoses of COPD will most likely have resting ABGs taken periodically. As lung function deteriorates over time with aging, resting ABGs show a worsening gas exchange capability and the $PO_2$ declines from the normal 96. It does not desaturate hemoglobin significantly until it reaches about 60. At present, ear or finger oximetry is being used more and more, as it is a quick, noninvasive, and quite satisfactory way of showing hemoglobin saturation. Currently, 85 percent saturation is considered the borderline value for the requirement of supplemental oxygen. Sometimes resting values are within normal range, but patients show desaturation with exercise. It is valuable to include exercise ABGs or oximetry to determine who would and who would not benefit from low-flow oxygen support during exercise. By elevating the inspired oxygen fraction ($FIO_2$), oxidative metabolism is supported and a higher exertional level may be reached before the anaerobic threshold appears. This permits a patient much more functional possibilities, and in critically ill patients the added support may be needed for brain, kidney, or heart metabolism.

Medicines taken for chronic pulmonary diseases tend to be for symptom relief rather than for cure. Breathlessness is the primary symptom, and congestion with secretion retention may be a component. Relief of breathlessness will depend upon the cause.

## Bronchodilators

Pharmacologic management of bronchospasm operates on the autonomic nervous system control of smooth muscle in the bronchiolar walls. These smooth muscles relax (causing bronchodilation) both through removal of cholinergic (parasympathetic) influence and by stimulation of adrenergic (sympathetic) receptors with norepinephrine, which actively results in bronchodilation. Thus, drugs of one group block cholinergic action and are called *parasympatholytic* drugs; they are atropine and the methylxanthines (theophylline or aminophylline) (Table 5.4). Drugs of the other group stimulate active relaxation of smooth muscle via sympathetic activation; they are called *sympathomimetics*. This group includes epinephrine, isoproterenol, isoetharine, metaproterenol sulfate, terbutaline sulfate, and albuterol (see Table 5.5).

Some but not all COPD patients have a bronchospastic component to their breathlessness complaint. When standard PFTs are measured, they are

**Table 5.4 Methylxanthines**

| Generic Drug | Trade Name | Primary Action | Side Effects |
|---|---|---|---|
| Theophylline | Theo-Dur<br>Slo-Phyllin<br>Elixophyllin<br>Aerolate<br>Fleet theophylline | Block cholinergic<br>stimulation with<br>passive relaxation<br>of bronchioles | Tachycardia<br>Palpitations<br>Arrhythmias<br>Hypertension<br>    or hypotension<br>Shock<br>Anxiety<br>Irritability<br>Fainting<br>Dizziness<br>Seizures<br>Indigestion<br>Diarrhea<br>Abdominal pain |
| Aminophylline | Aminodur Dura-Tabs<br>Aminophylline<br>    suppositories<br>Aminophylline ampule | Block cholinergic<br>stimulation with<br>passive relaxation<br>of bronchioles | Same as above |
| Oxtriphylline | Choledyl | Same as above | Same as above |

(Adapted from Zadai C: Pulmonary Pharmacology. In Malone T, Zimmerman J (eds): Drug Implications in the Rehabilitation Professions. JB Lippincott, Philadelphia, in press.)

**Table 5.5 Sympathomimetics**

| Generic Drug | Trade Name | Primary Action | Side Effects |
|---|---|---|---|
| Epinephrine | Adrenalin | Active bronchodilation | Tachycardia<br>Palpitations<br>Increased BP<br>Headache<br>Nervousness<br>Muscle tremor |
| Isoproterenol | Isuprel | Active bronchodilation | Tachycardia<br>Initial hypertension<br>Palpitations |
| Isoetharine | Bronkosol | Active bronchodilation | Tachycardia<br>Increased BP<br>Skeletal muscle tremor |
| Metaproterenol | Alupent<br>Metaprel | Active bronchodilation | Tachycardia<br>Hypertension<br>Muscle tremor |
| Terbutaline | Bricaryl<br>Brethine | Active bronchdilation | Muscle tremor<br>Less hypertension<br>Less tachycardia |
| Albuterol | Proventil<br>Ventolin | Active bronchodilation | Muscle tremor<br>Less tachycardia<br>Less hypertension |

(Adapted from Zadai C: Pulmonary Pharmacology. In Malone T, Zimmerman J (eds): Drug Implications in the Rehabilitation Professions. JB Lippincott, Philadelphia, in press.)

Table 5.6 Corticosteroids

| Generic Name | Trade Name | Primary Action | Side Effects |
|---|---|---|---|
| Hydrocortisone | Cortisol Cortef | Anti-inflammatory | Electrolyte disturbance Cushingoid syndrome with prolonged use |
| Prednisone | Prednisone | Same as above | Same as above Osteoporosis Peripheral neuropathies Myopathies |
| Prednisolone | Prednisolone | Same as above | Same as above |
| Methylprednisolone | Medrol | Same as above | Minimal side effects |
| Betamethasone | | Same as above | Same as above Can develop candidiasis with aerosol use |
| Dexamethasone | Decadron | Same as above | Same as above |
| Beclomethasone | Vanceril Beclovent | Same as above | Minimal side effects Hoarseness Candidiasis |

(Adapted from Zadai C: Pulmonary Pharmocology. In Malone T, Zimmerman J (eds): Drug Implications in the Rehabilitation Professions. JB Lippincott, Philadelphia, in press.)

first reported without bronchodilators; then an inhaled variety is adminis-tered, and a repeat PFT value is taken to determine whether the broncho-dilator improves air flow characteristics. Those patients who show signifi-cant improvement may be prescribed one form of bronchodilator.

### Anti-inflammatory Agents

Anti-inflammatory agents specific to pulmonary diseases are found to be useful symptomatic control drugs in asthma, bronchitis, bronchiectasis, pneumonia, and in some cases emphysema. These drugs are cromolyn so-dium and steroids (see Table 5.6).

Prednisone is administered orally, and Beclovent is an inhaled form of steroid. Steroids are indicated with long-term bronchospasm especially for patients in whom standard bronchospasm therapy does not totally relieve breathlessness. Patients with severe asthma or with chronic bronchitis and asthma are often the ones who require steroids. As an anti-inflammatory agent steroids help to reduce the processes that provoke smooth muscle swelling in bronchioles. Smooth muscles are permitted to relax and wheezing is reduced. There are many negative side effects associated with long-term steroidal therapy, and its systemic use over long periods is therefore avoided as much as possible.

### Antibiotics

When patients who have COPD show signs of an upper respiratory infection (e.g., color changes in sputum, odorous sputum, temperature elevation, feel-ing of malaise, and unusually severe shortness of breath), antibiotic therapy is essential. Some severe COPD patients will be on a low dose of antibiotic

Table 5.7 Antibiotics

| Generic Name | Trade Name | Primary Action | Side Effects |
|---|---|---|---|
| Penicillin | Penicillin G<br>Penicillin V<br>Oxacillin<br>Cloxacillin<br>Methacillin<br>Ampicillin<br>Amoxicillin<br>Carbenicillin | Inhibits cell wall<br>synthesis<br>Bactericidal | Can kill off competing<br>organisms and<br>promote growth of<br>resistant strains<br>Allergic reactions |
| Cephalosporin | Keflex<br>Keflin<br>Loridine<br>Velosef<br>Kafocin | Same as above | Nephrotoxicity with<br>tubular necrosis |
| Aminoglycosides | Streptomycin<br>Gentamicin<br>Tobramycin<br>Kanamycin<br>Amikacin<br>Neomycin | Interferes with<br>bacteria's protein<br>synthesis<br>Bactericidal | Ototoxicity<br>Neuromuscular<br>impairment<br>Renal tubular<br>Damage |
| Erythromycin | | Bacteriostatic | Few |
| Tetracycline | Tetracycline<br>Oxytetracycline<br>Chlortetracycline<br>Methacycline<br>Doxycycline | Bacteriostatic, by<br>interfering with<br>protein synthesis | GI irritation<br>Bone marrow<br>depression<br>Allergic responses |

(Adapted from Zadai C: Pulmonary Pharmocology. In Malone T, Zimmerman J (eds): Drug Implications in the Rehabilitation Professions. JB Lippincott, Philadelphia, in press.)

chronically; others will be given a standing prescription to be filled when they begin to feel symptomatic. For acute infectious processes, curative drugs are used to kill or inhibit microorganisms. These are bactericidal or bacteriostatic and include penicillin, cephalosporins, aminoglycosides, and tetracycline[8] (Table 5.7).

## Diuretics

Patients who have CHF, although compensated, can easily be thrown into worsening failure by too much exercise stress for the impaired myocardium to deal with. When the left ventricle fails, breathlessness is the most obvious symptom. It is accompanied by bibasilar rales and appearance of S3 and S4 heart sounds. Diuretic therapy reduces the circulating fluid by activating kidney function to a higher level, thus hemoconcentrating and reducing the fluid load on the right and left ventricles. Patients with COPD are more likely to first have right ventricular failure due to pulmonary congestion, but ultimately both ventricles typically develop CHF. If right ventricular failure develops, the usual signs and symptoms are weight gain, ankle edema, and jugular venous distention. (See Tables 4.3, 4.6, and 4.7).

## Expectorants

Patients for whom expectorants are prescribed are those who have difficulty clearing secretions. Rhonchi provide a clear breath-sound indication that secretions are present. This means they have a poor, ineffective cough, such as that of quadriplegics, or their sputum is remarkably thick and copious (see Ch. 10).

## Anticoagulants

Patients who have right ventricular dysfunction often develop supraventricular dysrhythmias such as atrial fibrillation. These patients are placed on anticoagulants to avoid potential problems of pulmonary embolism or cerebrovascular accident. (See Chapter 4.)

## Adjunct Equipment

### Air Compressor

An air compressor is an electrical device that compresses air, which then drives medication, with or without humidity added, into a steam or vaporous condition. This is inhaled for effective administration of a medication.

### Ventilator

A ventilator is used for the intubated patient, either via tracheostomy or via endotracheal tube, and provides the function of moving air in to the lungs because the muscles of ventilation are too weak or too nonfunctional to do an adequate job.

# Rehabilitation

Because breathlessness is such a terrifying experience for many patients, any activity that provokes the sensation is avoided. As activities are avoided, the vicious cycle is set up in which the functional capacity to perform activities once attempted is lost. Rehabilitation should aim to prevent this cycle and retard the inevitable decline of function as much as possible through a three-pronged approach.

## Emotional Support

It is helpful to deal with the guilt of long years of smoking (usually), and the fear of suffocating, and the humiliation of not being able to perform the usual activities of daily living (ADL). Patients who cope well with these issues can help those who are unable to. Many patients become very depressed because they cannot cope well. Group support and leadership by a trained health care provider are often a part of a rehabilitation program.

### Education

Education is important to patients who experience breathlessness. This education should cover the disease, medications, nutrition, breathing retraining (including pulmonary hygiene and paced breathing techniques), relaxation techniques and stress management, and exercise benefits and ways to perform exercise properly without undue breathlessness.

### Exercise

Aerobic exercise as a therapy for dyspnea is a component of a pulmonary rehabilitation program. Improvement in functional capacity in the population of patients with breathlessness may depend upon the achievement of an aerobic conditioning effect, either central (cardiac or pulmonary) or peripheral (cellular adaptations in working muscles). It may depend upon the psychological conditioning of the patient to tolerate the sensation of breathlessness without panic. It may depend upon a learning effect or a local strengthening or endurance training effect of the diaphragm muscle and/or other muscles of ventilation with a consequent improvement in the pattern of use of these muscles with exercise.

The results of 8 weeks of daily exercises using walking, bicycling exercise, upper body cranking, wall pulleys, and stair climbing show remarkable functional improvement as reported by patients and as measured objectively on several functional tests (see physical therapy evaluation for the 6-minute walk test). The repeat performances of patients who undergo the incremental continuous exercise test at work rate increments of 4 Watts for those with severe COPD, 6 or 12 W for less severe cases, and 25 W for other patients do not show improvements of primary ventilatory exercise measures, nor do the patients increase their peak $\dot{V}O_2$. However, they do perform longer and to higher intensities before they reach their peak $\dot{V}O_2$ and maximum minute ventilation (max $\dot{V}E$). Their ratio of max$\dot{V}E$ to MVV is often improved, showing a greater ventilatory reserve than prior to the rehabilitation program (unpublished data) (see section on PFTs). These objective changes do not explain adequately the functional capacity improvements found in nearly all COPD patients who undergo a rehabilitation program. Therefore, psychological and other physiologic mechanisms may be contributing to their improvement.

## Invasive Monitoring

See Chapter 4 for descriptions of Swan-Ganz catheterization and arterial lines.

## Invasive Procedures

### Bronchoscopy and Pulmonary Lavage

In cases in which foreign substances block airways or lung tumors or secretions obstruct the flow of air, a bronchial lavage via bronchoscopy may be done. A fine brush is passed through the fiberoptic tube under local anesthesia into the area of obstruction. A sweep of the airways can provide a sample of tissue or secretions for analysis as well as help to clear the smaller bronchi with the aid of suction. For a complete discussion of complications and risks from this procedure see the discussion of Bronchoscopy under Tests earlier in this chapter.

## Chest Tube

In the case of pneumothorax producing breathlessness, a chest tube is inserted into the chest cavity to suction out the air that has collapsed the lung. With the provision of suction, a negative pressure may be restored, which will re-expand the collapsed lung. As long as air remains within the pleural cavity, the positive pressure created by this air impinges upon the lung and keeps it collapsed. A chest tube may be maintained for a long period of weeks or even months or until re-expansion is achieved and the tube can be withdrawn gradually without introduction of more air into the pleural space. Once a tube is withdrawn and a healed seal is demonstrated, a patient should be free to begin usual activities.

## Intra-aortic Balloon Pump

In patients with CHF, a balloon, which can be inflated and deflated in a regular cycle by an external pump, is often placed in the femoral artery. This action assists the heart in its primary job of circulating blood around the systematic circulation system and thereby gives the heart a rest. For the failing heart such a rest can be of great benefit. Patients are usually not on the intra-aortic balloon pump (IABP) for a very long period, as they either go to surgery or are controlled with drugs such as digitalis to prevent decompensation of their heart failure (See Ch. 4).

## Mechanical Ventilation

For patients who develop respiratory failure and thus experience severe dyspnea at rest, mechanical ventilation may be indicated, and the invasive procedure preceding this is intubation. An endotracheal tube is passed via either the mouth or nostril into the trachea and the mechanical ventilator tubing then connects directly to this tube. An endotracheal tube is usually considered a temporary measure. For patients who require longer-term mechanical ventilation, a tracheostomy is performed for the connection. This requires a puncture of the trachea at a level just over the cricoid membrane.

The mechanical ventilator provides the function of moving air into the lungs, which is normally carried out by the musculoskeletal pump. Adjustments of partial pressures of gases may enhance gas exchange as well.

Patients on ventilators can be mobilized to perform certain functional activities as well as exercise programs. There may be reason to believe that difficult-to-wean patients may do better during a weaning program if they are mobilized while on the ventilator.[9]

Some forms that exercise may take include supine cycling using a restorator, stationary bicycling, and marching in place, all while the mechanical ventilator continues to operate for the patient. Alternatively, a second helper can use an ambu bag on the patient during exercise off the ventilator. If a patient is on a weaning program, this whole body exercise should be performed while the patient is fully mechanically ventilated rather than during or just after a period of weaning, when the ventilatory muscles are most fatigued. The principle of conservation of energy should be employed in these critically ill patients.

## PHYSICAL THERAPY INTERVENTION

## Interview

Key questions to add to the general physical therapy interview about this complaint of breathlessness are:

1.  When you get short of breath do you gag? Do you panic?
2.  What do you do to get relief when you feel short of breath?
3.  What conditions or activities bring on shortness of breath?
4.  Do you cough when you get short of breath?
5.  Why do you think you get breathless?

## Physical Therapy Evaluation

For a synopsis of findings using specific evaluation procedures listed for musculoskeletal and cardiopulmonary areas, see Table 5.8.

### Functional Evaluation

As a part of the physical therapy evaluation a 12- or a 6-minute walk test has become an extremely valuable functional evaluation tool, especially in patients whose main symptom is dyspnea. This is a test in which the distance a patient is able to walk continuously in 12 minutes is the major measurement of endurance. It is also useful to take pre- and postwalk measures of heart rate, respiratory rate, and blood pressure. The patient must be told to assume the pace that will require his maximal effort, yet will permit him to continue walking for the whole duration of the test. A 6-minute walk test is a modified version, sometimes easier for patients to perform. Patients who are wheelchair-bound can do this test in their chairs. In addition, other functional activities, if sufficiently standardized so that they may easily be repeated,

**Table 5.8 Physical Therapy Evaluation of Breathlessness**

| Procedure | Pathology | | |
|---|---|---|---|
| | CHF | COPD | Restrictive |
| Musculoskeletal | | | |
| Posture evaluation | — | Barrel chest<br>Stiff ribs<br>Forward head<br>Elevated shoulders | Kyphosis<br>Scoliosis<br>Obesity |
| Range of motion | — | Shoulder range of motion<br>Trunk mobility<br>Neck mobility | Trunk mobility<br>Neck mobility |
| Manual muscle test | — | Abdominal muscle strength | — |
| Cardiopulmonary:<br>Inspection | Jugular vein distension<br>Cardiac apical pulsations | Accessory muscle use<br>Symmetrical thoracic excursion, inspiration/expiration ratio<br>Paradoxical abdominal motion<br>Purse-lip breathing<br>Color, general appearance "pink puffer" vs. "blue bloater"<br>Clubbing | Spinal deformity |
| Palpation | Point of maximal impulse<br>Chest pain for trigger points<br>Peripheral pulses<br>Edema | Inspiration/expiration excursion | — |

(Continued)

**Table 5.8 Physical Therapy Evaluation of Breathlessness** (*Continued*)

| Procedure | CHF | Pathology COPD | Restrictive |
|---|---|---|---|
| | | Pathology | |
| Percussion | — | Resonance | Consolidation Dull-thud |
| Auscultation | S3, S4 Bibasilar rales, symmetrical | Decreased breath sounds Rhonchi Wheezes Rales | Decreased breath sounds Rhonchi Wheezes Rales |
| Cough | Yes Productive, frothy foamy, secretions | Yes or no Mucoid Green, yellow, tan, white | Yes or no Mucoid |
| Vital Signs | | | |
| Blood pressure | Low | Normal or high due to drugs or age | Normal |
| Heart rate | High, compensatory tachycardia | High with methylxanthine drugs | Normal |
| Heart rhythm | Normal sinus Premature atrial contractions | Premature atrial contractions Atrial fibrillation | Normal sinus |
| Respiratory rate | High | High | High |
| Temperature | Normal | Normal | Normal |
| O$_2$ saturation, rest | Normal | Low | Low |
| O$_2$ saturation, exercise | Normal | Can desaturate | Can desaturate |

may be used. Thus, two flights of stairs, taken at a constant speed as with a metronome, may be used—or even one flight for a lower functional level.

Bicycle ergometry protocols have been developed for evaluation of dyspnea (See discussion of $\dot{V}O_2$ stress testing above).

Treadmill evaluations may be valuable for patients with breathlessness. A slow walking pace for a long duration during which the pace itself is enforced provides a consistent power output. The response to this, in terms of oxygen consumption and ventilatory and cardiac responses, provides the necessary dose-response information for the physical therapist to use in designing an exercise prescription for the patient's rehabilitation program. Dynamic exercise that mobilizes the oxygen transport system, permits free breathing, but remains at an intensity below the symptomatic threshold for dyspnea will place an aerobic stimulus upon the physiologic systems involved in exercise without recruiting the anaerobic pathways that would lead to ventilatory inadequacy. (See discussion of $\dot{V}O_2$ exercise testing.)

In order to aim for functional improvement, exercise is usually prescribed to include:

1. Large muscle mass—legs, trunk, shoulder girdle
2. Specific inspiratory muscle training
3. Daily 10- to 20-minute exercise bouts (longer if tolerated)
4. Borg scale adapted to dyspnea sensation, intensity to 13 or 14 (see Table 6.2)
5. Pre-exercise stretches, breathing exercises, 15 minutes
6. Postexercise cool-down, 10 minutes

# REFERENCES

1. Wasserman K: Dyspnea on exertion. Is it the heart or the lungs? JAMA 248:2039, 1982
2. Wasserman K, Whipp B: Exercise physiology in health and disease. Am Rev Respir Dis 112:219, 1975
3. Åstrand P, Rohdal A: Textbook of Work Physiology. 3rd Ed. McGraw-Hill, New York, 1986
4. Shapiro B, Harrison R, Trout C: Clinical Applications of Respiratory Care. Year Book Medical Publishers, Chicago, 1977
5. Dreisin RB, Albert RK, Talley PA, et al: Flexible fiberoptic bronchoscopy in the teaching hospital. Yield and complications. Chest 74:144, 1978
6. Pereira W, Kovnat DM, Snider GL: A prospective cooperative study of complications following flexible fiberoptic bronchoscopy. Chest 73:813, 1978
7. Suratt PM, Smiddy JF, Gruber B: Deaths and complications associated with fiberoptic bronchoscopy. Chest 69:747, 1976

8. Zadai C: Pulmonary Pharmacology. In Malone T, Zimmerman J (eds): Drug Implications in the Rehabilitation Professions. JB Lippincott, Philadelphia, in press
9. Holtackers T: Rehabilitation of the ventilator dependent patient. Mayo Clinic Special Interest paper. Am. Phys. Ther. Assoc. Feb 5, 1984

## SUGGESTED READINGS

Cash J (ed): Chest, Heart, and Vascular Disorders for Physiotherapists. Faber & Faber, London, 1975

Irwin S, Tecklin J: Cardiopulmonary Physical Therapy. CV Moxby, St. Louis, 1985

Shayevitz M, Shayevitz B: Living Well with Emphysema and Bronchitis. Doubleday, New York, 1985

Webber C, Janecki J: Cardiopulmonary Exercise Testing. Physiologic Principles and General Applications. WB Saunders, Philadelphia, 1986

West J: Respiratory Physiology. Williams & Wilkins, Baltimore, 1979

West J: Respiratory Pathophysiology. Williams & Wilkins, Baltimore, 1979

# FATIGUE

# 6

Fatigue becomes a symptom of concern when it occurs in a patient with minimal provocation. Very low level exertion should not evoke fatigue unless there is a pathologic process undermining the available energy sources or the body's ability to use fuel substrates. For the purpose of this chapter we do not refer to fatigue as the state of sleep deprivation but rather as the loss of or lack of energy with which to perform a reasonable level of activity. Table 6.1 identifies a variety of causes of fatigue.

## CHART REVIEW

Because fatigue sources may be neurologic, muscular, metabolic, cardiac, or pulmonary, a patient history is a very important source of information. In addition, numerous tests may enlighten us about the fatigue problem, and a chart review to ascertain what tests have been done could yield all the necessary information to sort out our patient's problem.

### Medical History

On the chart it is unlikely that the medical history will report any specific findings on fatigue. Information about fatigue can be obtained indirectly by looking for the answers to many of the following questions.

Is the fatigue sensation a local or a generalized phenomenon? Local muscular fatigue will be described as heaviness, ache, and a dull sense of pain, occasionally accompanied by muscular cramp. General fatigue is commonly described as inability or unwillingness to keep going, a distinct need to rest, and a very diffuse sensation.

Next, what provokes the sense of fatigue in question? When does the patient experience this fatigue? What triggers the sensation? Is there a fairly consistent level of exertion that provokes the sensation? Is it correlated with any particular activity or with any other person, object, or site? What are associated symptoms, if any—for example, shortness of breath, pain in the chest, sense of palpitations, or headache. Given the medical diagnosis of

**Table 6.1 Differential Diagnosis of Fatigue**

| Possible Causes | Possible Findings | Stimuli | Pathology |
|---|---|---|---|
| Local muscle glycogen depletion | "The wall"; lack of whole body energy | Endurance exercise of long duration | None |
| Lactate accumulation in muscle and blood | Hyperventilation; breathlessness; loss of motivation | Deconditioning<br>Anaerobic metabolism<br>Organ ischemia<br>Breath-holding activities | None |
| Poor motivation | Apathy; lethargy; may have pain in muscles | Overuse of muscles<br>Depression<br>Anxiety<br>Drugs | Chemical imbalances in the brain (?) |
| Calcium ion depletion | Tetanus; muscle cramping; muscle pain | Prolonged use of muscle<br>Electrical stimulation | None |
| Low cardiac output | Inotropic incompetence; low blood pressure; increased HR; pallor; frequent ventricular ectopy | Age<br>Deconditioning<br>Microbes<br>Alcoholism | Coronary artery disease<br>Aortic valve dysfunction<br>Cardiomyopathy<br>Myocarditis |

| Anemia | General body fatigue; loss of energy; low hematocrit | Blood loss<br>Cardiopulmonary bypass machine<br>Dietary<br>Deconditioning<br>Genetic | Neoplasm<br>Sickle cell<br>Pernicious<br>Iron deficiency |
|---|---|---|---|
| Dehydration | Dry mouth; general loss of energy; low BP; increased HR | Diarrhea<br>Vomiting<br>Heat exposure<br>Fever<br>Blood loss | Cholera<br>GI bleeding<br>Infection<br>GI irritation |
| Hypothyroidism | Lethargy; dull, slow speech; slow movements | Genetic (?) | Thyroid gland dysfunction |
| Hypoxia | $PO_2 < 55$ mmHg; $O_2$ saturation <85%; cyanosis; increased RR; increased HR; pallor; breathlessness; stupor; lightheadedness | Exercise<br>Apnea<br>Hypoventilation | Respiratory failure<br>Pulmonary embolus<br>Arteriovenous shunt of heart or lungs |
| Hyperglycemia | Increased hemoglobin A1c; ketone breath; ketone bodies in urine; high blood sugar | High blood sugar | Diabetes mellitus with insulin deficiency |

the patient, do the accompanying symptoms make sense? What is the influence of rest and body position on the symptom? Leaning forward on the forearms is commonly seen in patients with chronic obstructive pulmonary disease (COPD). When did the patient first begin to notice the problem of fatigue as now experienced? What medical diagnoses does the patient have? Does the medical history help determine what system is primarily involved in fatigue?

### Implications for Physical Therapy

1.  If there is a cardiac diagnosis, such as coronary artery disease (CAD) or congestive heart failure (CHF), look for the results of an exercise tolerance test (ETT) in the medical record. Other tests may help determine the extent of myocardial dysfunction: A gated blood pool study (GBPS), an echocardiogram, a cardiac catheterization. Be prepared to monitor such a patient for heart rate (HR), and blood pressure (BP), and by electrocardiography (ECG) (rhythm strip).
2.  If there is a pulmonary diagnosis, such as emphysema, asthma, chronic bronchitis, sarcoidosis, or pulmonary fibrosis, look for the results of pulmonary function tests (PFTs) and a chest x-ray to determine the severity of the problem. Blood tests such as arterial blood gas (ABG) determinations may have been made to determine the need for supplemental $O_2$. There may even be a $\dot{V}O_2$ exercise test to determine whether cardiac or pulmonary disease limits the patient more. Check for breath sounds in the physical examination done by the physician. Adventitious sounds should be checked each time prior to beginning physical therapy treatment to determine the need for specific breathing exercises or pulmonary hygiene.
3.  If the patient is diabetic, check for the hemoglobin A1c, which will determine the adequacy of glucose metabolic control over a 2- to 3-month period. If this runs low, the patient may experience fatigue from hypoglycemia and would obtain most benefit from provision of supplemental sugar acutely, with further nutritional follow-up suggested. If hemoglobin A1c runs high, either the medication schedule needs to be changed to better accommodate to demands of exercise, or the diet should be altered, and for this a phone call to the patient's dietician or physician may be helpful.
4.  If the patient is hypothyroid, check the T3, T4 blood test to see if more hormone supplement is needed.
5.  Check hematocrit to see if the patient is anemic. Dietary support should gradually reduce fatigue from this source.

## Physical Examination

### Vital Signs

To help determine whether there is an immediate cardiopulmonary cause of a patient's fatigue, the following vital signs should be recorded.

## Heart Rate

Low cardiac output, local muscle glycogen depletion, lactate accumulation, and anemia could all produce an elevation of HR with fatigue. Low HR would accompany hypothyroidism.

## Blood Pressure

Blood pressure is low at rest or in response to exercise in a low cardiac output state, such as in CHF or cardiomyopathy with fatigue.

## Respiratory Rate

Respiratory rate (RR) is elevated in lung disease and in CHF. If the RR is high but the cardiac variables appear to be normal, the patient may be in an anxiety state with hyperventilation or may have serious COPD, which should be documented in his chart. If the cause of fatigue is CHF, the patient will be hypotensive and tachycardic, will show pallor, and may have ventricular dysrhythmias.

## Auscultation

If there is reason to suspect CHF as the cause of fatigue, auscultation will detect rales in both lung bases, perhaps wheezes, and the presence of S3, S4, or both sounds.

# Tests

Fatigue can be the single consequence of a multiplicity of problems. For example, the diabetic patient who has poorly controlled diabetes may also have atherosclerotic peripheral artery disease and/or CAD and therefore will suffer unusual fatigue from the combined effects of the various disease states. It is therefore useful to look for a variety of medical tests in the patient's chart. The tests discussed below are examples.

## Laboratory Values

### Blood Glucose

Elevations in blood glucose and/or hemoglobin A1c results may be labeled as a diabetic response and could help account for one source of fatigue, which would be experienced as a generalized, diffuse sense of fatigue (see Ch. 8).

**Implications for Physical Therapy.** A source of sugar should be ready if the patient will be exercising. A finger stick glucometer may be a useful instrument to have available during treatment.

## Arterial Blood Gases

Arterial blood gases will provide many important pieces of information about the patient's metabolism. First, if the pH is below 7.4, the patient is acidotic. It may be a respiratory acidosis, as seen if the $PCO_2$ is above 40 mmHg, or it may be a metabolic acidosis if the bicarbonate ion concentration is above 24 mM/L. Acidosis from whatever cause is usually accompanied by general body fatigue. Patients may be acidotic owing to lactic acid accumulation when there is insufficient oxygen to support an activity or during isometric activities that are sustained. Patients may be acidotic owing to inability to "blow off" sufficient $CO_2$ to balance the metabolic equation. This is likely due to inadequate breathing. Does the patient have COPD? Does he have sleep apnea or any other sort of apnea? Is he Pickwickian? A blood lactate test (below) will help in the differential diagnosis. If the pH is above 7.4, the patient is alkalotic. A respiratory alkalosis is found if the $PCO_2$ is below 40. This is associated with lightheadedness and loss of consciousness due to hyperventilation. A metabolic alkalosis exists if the bicarbonate ion level is below 24. This situation may generate extreme fatigue and could indicate kidney failure.

**Implications for Physical Therapy**
Check $PO_2$ to determine need for supplemental $O_2$.
Correlate RR with $PCO_2$ to determine whether patient is breathless, and if so, how severe this condition is.
Check pH to determine metabolic state.

## Blood Lactate

The normal blood lactate value is 0.6 to 1.8 mEq/L. A high blood lactate correlates with a low pH, signifying metabolic acidosis. Any elevation may help to explain general body fatigue. Some people especially athletes, tolerate unusually high values; however, most people experience extreme fatigue and loss of motivation with lactate accumulation.

**Implications for Physical Therapy.** Metabolic acidosis indicates insufficient $O_2$ to support aerobic metabolism. Consider the reasons, and decide if supplemental $O_2$ will help. Use of the ear or finger oximeter will provide definitive evidence that $O_2$ should be given. An $O_2$ saturation that drops below 85 percent should indicate the need for supplemental $O_2$.

## Blood Enzymes and Isoenzymes

Serial blood studies are done as a way of marking the necrosis of a body tissue and the extent of damage. As discussed in Chapter 4, the CPK-MB fraction is a specific myocardial isoenzyme and CPK-MM is skeletal muscle-specific. These elevated levels will not produce fatigue in themselves, but would indicate muscle damage which would be expected to produce fatigue, or pain. When the myocardium is damaged, as in a myocardial infarction there is such an insult to the pump that an acute recovery period can be marked by low cardiac output. The more extensive the damage and the greater the number of such insults, the more intense is the fatigue.

**Implications for Physical Therapy**

If the MB band is elevated, there is clear evidence of myocardial damage, and ECG monitoring should be done.

Measures of HR and BP are critical in such a patient.

## Complete Blood Count and Electrolytes

A complete blood count will yield valuable information for sorting out the source of the patient's fatigue. Anemia, or low hemoglobin, and low hematocrit will indicate a reduction of the oxygen-carrying capacity of the blood, which limits the metabolic supply of aerobically derived energy. An elevated white cell count indicates infection, which means that the body's energy is already at a high level in an effort to fight off an invading organism. Electrolyte levels will help us determine whether the normal balance is off. Low potassium and high potassium levels are both causes of fatigue due to disturbances in membrane potentials, and frequently potassium ion shifts result in cardiac dysrhythmias. Calcium ions are required to trigger muscular contraction. If these are in low supply, there is a local muscular fatigue potential, as well as myocardial contraction "fatigue." (See table in Appendix for normal values.)

**Implications for Physical Therapy**

Low calcium ion usually causes muscle twitches and can bring on a tetanus. Do not exercise.

Potassium ion disturbance means the patient should be monitored for subsequent dysrhythmias after medical intervention has occurred.

If white blood cells are elevated, check for fever, look for chest x-ray, and check sputum for sign of systemic infection or upper respiratory tract infection. Dysrhythmias can be generated by bacterial endocarditis or myocarditis.

Anemia can be reversed with diet or iron supplement over time. Exercise should be of low intensity, probably aerobic at less than 60 percent of maximum HR with planned rests. Teach patient to pace activity with rests.

## Thyroid Function Test

The thyroid function as determined by the T3/T4 test should help to determine if hypothyroidism may be an explanation of fatigue. If the thyroid output is insufficient, the metabolic rate does not rise appropriately, and simple supplementation with a thyroid derivative hormone can reverse the fatigue symptom dramatically.

## Exercise Tolerance Test

An exercise treadmill test, using a standard procedure such as the Bruce protocol, helps to determine whether the heart is implicated in fatigue. A poor duration of the test shows early fatigue, appearance of cardiac symptoms, or both. Failure of the BP to rise with increasing work loads indicates inadequate cardiac output to meet the demands of the exercise. A maximal oxygen consumption measurement indicates a patient's aerobic capacity, which, if low, helps to account for poor exercise tolerance on the basis of deconditioning (see Ch. 5).

## Cardiac Catheterization

In low cardiac output states such as that found in CHF, an actual measure of cardiac output done in the catheterization laboratory will help to determine the significance of this finding for the patient's functional potential (see Ch. 4). When the ejection fraction (EF) and cardiac output are low, ventricular disfunction may be the direct cause of general body fatigue.

**Implications for Physical Therapy**
A low EF, less than 40 percent, indicates depressed ventricular function. Keep track of HR, BP, symptoms, and ECG.
Progress activity program gradually; the lower the EF, the more gradual the progression.

## Muscle Biopsy

A muscle biopsy needle may be employed to obtain a sample of muscle fibers for histochemical analysis in order to diagnose certain rare muscle diseases that result in persistent local muscle fatigue and soreness. It would identify primary muscle wasting diseases such as the muscular dystrophies or metabolic disorders such as McArdle's syndrome, in which a phosphorylation enzyme is absent.

## Electromyography

Electromyography is done with needle electrodes as a diagnostic test when neuromuscular diseases are suspected as a cause of fatigue. Abnormal findings that correlate with local muscle fatigue are fasciculations rather than normal action potentials.

**Implications for Physical Therapy**
Genetic metabolic disorders and neuromuscular diseases are irreversible, and exercise will not reverse fatigue symptoms.
Expect fatigue to worsen slowly over time with progressive muscle wasting diseases such as muscular dystrophy.

## MEDICAL-SURGICAL INTERVENTION

### Pharmacology

Drug treatment of fatigue depends entirely upon the diagnosis because so many different medical conditions can produce fatigue as one of several or many complaints. Treatment of the underlying problem will reverse the fatigue but not prevent usual expected fatigue from reappearing. Examples of treatment for fatigue include an iron supplement for anemia, thyroid hormone supplement for hypothyroidism, glucose for hypoglycemia, oxygen therapy for pulmonary dysfunction, digitalis to enhance cardiac contractility, and Elavil for mood elevation.

It is perhaps worth noting that certain medications prescribed for cardiac problems and psychogenic problems can cause unusual fatigue symptoms. Examples of these include β blockers and antidepressants.

### Rehabilitation

Often fatigability is reversible with a combination of pharmacologic intervention, emotional support, and exercise training. A vicious cycle may be quickly established in which patients who experience fatigue do less and less exercise and become increasingly deconditioned to a point at which attempting low level activities produces severe fatigue, shortness of breath, and possibly other symptoms as well. The unpleasantness of these sensations causes avoidance of all activities, which simply makes the problems worsen. Education about energy conservation techniques and pacing of activities to avoid lactate buildup may be helpful. A paced exercise intervention program and emotional support can be effective for people who have fatigue as a primary complaint (see Chs. 4 and 5).

In deconditioned patients aerobic training will result in improved physical working capacity, higher maximal $\dot{V}O_2$, and much less fatigability. With a high degree of training, glycogen sparing in muscles and increased lactate tolerance delay the onset of fatigue dramatically (see Ch. 5).

### Invasive Monitoring

The major implication for invasive monitoring when fatigue is the primary complaint is the possibility of low cardiac output states. Swan-Ganz monitoring provides information regarding cardiac output and hemodynamic pressure levels. High pulmonary wedge pressure is a sign of pulmonary hypertension or pulmonary edema and suggests a pressure gradient for the right ventricle that can lead to right ventricular CHF over time and, soon thereafter, to inevitable left ventricular CHF. This will be associated with fatigue (see Ch. 4).

## Invasive Procedures

Invasive procedures are generally not indicated as treatments for fatigue. Rather, diagnostic conditions such as CHF, kidney failure, diabetes, and hypothyroidism may require invasive procedures such as catheterization, dialysis, or surgery. Therefore the reader is referred to other sections of this book and other medical texts on procedures for diagnostic categories.

## PHYSICAL THERAPY EVALUATION

The physical therapy evaluation should follow the generic guidelines found in Chapter 3.

## Interview

### Key Questions

Add these key questions to the generic physical therapy patient interview.

1. What does your fatigue feel like? (Sample answers: weak, cramps in muscles, sleepy, low energy, too relaxed, soreness, or pain.)
2. How well do you sleep?
3. What brings on your feeling of fatigue?
4. What do you do to get relief?
5. Do you ever get short of breath or dizzy or lose coordination with fatigue? (Answer may provide a clue to anxiety-provoked hyperventilation.)
6. Do you get unusually or frequently thirsty? (Diabetes will create thirst.)

## Evaluation

The measurements of muscular strength and endurance are critical in the evaluation of fatigue. If objective measurement of endurance (using the Cybex Fatigue Index, for example) is available, this should be the most specific, repeatable, and valid measure for the symptom of fatigue. The cardiopulmonary evaluation should emphasize the following techniques.

### Inspection

Check for paradoxical abdominal motion; this is a sign of fatigue of the diaphragm and is a poor breathing technique. The abdominal wall is sucked inwards during inspiration when it should bulge passively outwards as the abdominal contents are pushed out of the way of the diaphragm muscle's descent. Accessory muscle use may be visible.

**Table 6.2 Rating of Perceived Exertion Scale**

| 6 | No exertion at all |
|---|---|
| 7 | Extremely light |
| 8 | |
| 9 | Very light |
| 10 | |
| 11 | Light |
| 12 | |
| 13 | Somewhat hard |
| 14 | |
| 15 | Hard (heavy) |
| 16 | |
| 17 | Very hard |
| 18 | |
| 19 | Extremely hard |
| 20 | Maximal exertion |

(From Borg G: Perceived exertion as indicator of somatic stress. Scand J Rehabil Med 2:92, 1970.)

If CHF of the right ventricle is suspected, check for jugular venous distention, which would correlate with fatigue.

## Auscultation

If CHF is suspected, listen for all four heart sounds, and check both bases of the lungs for rales.

BP will be low if CHF is present.
HR will be high if CHF is present.
RR will be high if left ventricular CHF is present.

## Functional Assessment

### Endurance Assessment

Choose an activity that the patient can perform reliably and, given enough rest, repeatedly. Determine pace and total time with which he performs the activity. Take HR, RR, and BP before and after the activity. Listen to breath sounds before and after. Oximetry will be useful if you suspect poor oxygenation of the periphery. It is also often useful to use the rating-of-perceived-exertion scale created by Gunnar Borg to determine the patient's fatigue perception (Table 6.2). In many patients this value should correlate with their HR response to the activity by a factor of 10. As a rule of thumb, a rating of 13 indicates a reasonable training level of exertion for many patients. Above this rating they may be overexerting, and under this level they cannot achieve conditioning benefits. Since the rating scale is subjective, a 13 to 14 rating is relative and seems to be the most consistent point on the scale for a threshold level of tolerance that is also beneficial.[1,2]

## REFERENCES

1. Borg G: Perceived exertion as indicator of somatic stress. Scand J Rehabil Med 2:92, 1970
2. Smutok M, Skrinor G, Pandolf K: Exercise intensity: subjective regulation by perceived exertion. Arch Phys Med Rehabil 61:569, 1980

## SUGGESTED READINGS

Astrand P, Rohdal A: Textbook of Work Physiology, 3rd Ed. McGraw-Hill, New York, 1986

Felig P, Wahren J: Fuel Homeostasis in exercise. N Engl J Med 293:1078, 1975

Steggmann J: Exercise Physiology. Year Book Medical Publishers, Chicago, 1981

Wahren J, Hagenfeldt I, Felig P: Splanchnic and leg exchange of glucose, amino acids and free fatty acids during exercise in diabetes mellitus. J Clin Invest 55:1303, 1975

Webber C, Janecki J: Cardiopulmonary Exercise Testing and Physiologic Principles and Clinical Application. WB Saunders, Philadelphia, 1986

# IRREGULAR HEART BEAT

# 7

The presence of an irregular heart beat (dysrhythmia), confirmed by an electrocardiogram (ECG), can be a benign or extremely ominous finding. The purpose of this chapter is to assist the physical therapist to differentiate the severity of irregularities in pulse and to feel confident in working with patients who exhibit benign forms of irregular heart beat. Examples of heart rhythms and common predisposing conditions are found in Table 7.1 and Figures 7.1 through 7.9.

## CHART REVIEW

The management of an irregular heart beat ranges from no intervention to risky and life-threatening procedures. The strategy the physician decides to utilize with each patient becomes clear as findings from medical history, physical examination, and laboratory and diagnostic tests are known. Although the management of dysrhythmias can be controversial, generally therapy is directed at symptom relief and maintenance of cardiac output, thereby reducing morbidity and/or mortality.

### Medical History

The patient may recognize an abnormal sensation in the chest. This sensation may be described as a palpitation, fluttering, or pounding. Occasionally dysrhythmias, usually ventricular in origin, are described as a feeling that the heart is "flipping over" in the chest. There may be feelings of lightheadedness or dizziness associated with the abnormal sensation. When the pulse is palpated, it may feel rapid or irregular, as if the heart "skipped" a beat.

What is the duration of the sensation's presence, what brings it on, and what does the patient do for relief of the symptom? Some dysrhythmias, those typically generated from the atria, may be very subtle; the patient may

**Table 7.1 Differential Diagnosis of Irregular Heart Beat**

| Heart Rhythm | Possible Findings | Stimuli | Pathology |
|---|---|---|---|
| Atrial fibrillation | Irregularly irregular pulse; ventricular response rate variable | Myocardial ischemia<br>Digitalis toxicity<br>Atrial hypertrophy<br>Atrial flutter | COPD<br>CAD<br>Mitral stenosis<br>Aortic stenosis<br>Cardiomyopathy |
| Atrial flutter | Usually rapid, regular pulse; ventricular response rate constant; atrial rate >220 bpm Sawtooth pattern on ECG | Myocardial ischemia<br>Digitalis toxicity<br>Atrial hypertrophy | COPD<br>CAD<br>Atrioventricular valve disease<br>Cardiomyopathy |
| Paroxysmal atrial tachycardia (PAT) | Regular heart rate, 160–220 bpm; ventricular response rate constant; spontaneous onset and cessation of "palpitations" | Caffeine<br>High catecholamine state<br>Anxiety | Wolf-Parkinson-White syndrome |
| Premature atrial contractions (PACs) | Pause in pulse can be regular or irregular, occasional or frequent May be associated with HR 60–150 bpm | Caffeine<br>High catecholamine state<br>Anxiety<br>Atrial hypertrophy<br>Atrial ischemia | COPD<br>Mitral valve prolapse |
| Premature junctional contraction (PJC), premature nodal beat (PNB) | Pause can be regular or irregular, occasional or frequent Associated with HR 40–60 bpm Rare | AV node conduction abnormality<br>Failure of SA node | Sick sinus syndrome |

| | | | |
|---|---|---|---|
| Premature ventricular contraction (PVC), ventricular premature beat (VPB) | Feel skip in pulse<br>Pause can be regular or irregular, occasional or frequent | Conduction disturbance<br>Drugs<br>Spontaneous<br>Caffeine<br>High catecholamine state<br>Exercise<br>Anxiety<br>Myocardial ischemia<br>Failure of SA-AV nodes<br>Low potassium | "Athlete's heart"<br>COPD<br>CAD<br>Ventricular aneurysm<br>Sick sinus syndrome |
| Bigeminy | Feel a skip every second beat | Same as above | Same as above |
| Couplet | Feel a longer pause | Same as above | Same as above |
| Ventricular tachycardia | Decreased blood pressure<br>Lightheadedness | Same as above | Same as above |
| Pacemaker | Pause in pulse can be irregular or regular, can be rare or frequent<br>Paced beats may be among normal beats, or all beats may be paced<br>Pacing spike may be before or in the middle of the P wave or QRS complex | Bradycardia<br>Acute myocardial infarction | Sick sinus syndrome<br>Complete heart block<br>Conduction tissue ischemia |

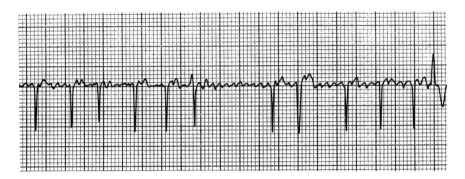

**Fig. 7.1** Atrial fibrillation

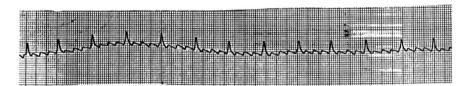

**Fig. 7.2** Atrial flutter

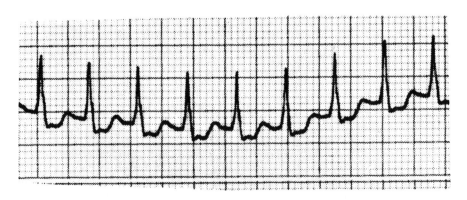

**Fig. 7.3** Paroxysmal atrial tachycardia (PAT)

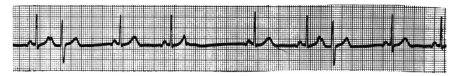

**Fig. 7.4** Premature atrial contractions (PACs).

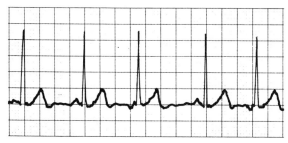

LEAD 2

**Fig. 7.5** Premature junctional contraction (PJC), premature nodal beat (PNB). (Reproduced from Advanced Cardiac Life Support, published by the American Heart Association, 1983. By permission of the American Heart Association Inc.)

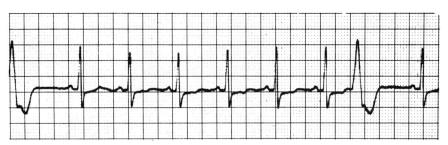

LEAD 2

**Fig. 7.6** Premature ventricular contraction (PVC), ventricular premature beat (VPB). (Reproduced from Advanced Cardiac Life Support, published by the American Heart Association, 1983. By permission of the American Heart Association Inc.)

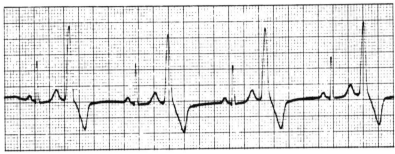

LEAD 2

**Fig. 7.7** Ventricular bigeminy. (Reproduced from Advanced Cardiac Life Support, published by the American Heart Association, 1983. By permission of the American Heart Association Inc.)

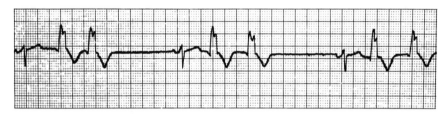

**Fig. 7.8** Couplet. (Reproduced from Advanced Cardiac Life Support, published by the American Heart Association, 1983. By permission of the American Heart Association Inc.)

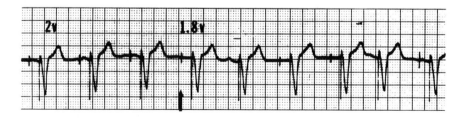

**Fig. 7.9** Pacemaker.

ignore them and may be vague as to their onset, duration, or relief. Does the sensation clearly occur after nicotine or caffeine ingestion, during anxiety, or with exercise? Does removal of the stimulus relieve the irregular heart beat in most instances? More ominous dysrhythmias, such as atrial or ventricular tachycardia or fibrillation, may only be terminated with medication, electrical cardioversion, or defibrillation.

The frequency and the length of time the dysrhythmia occurs are important factors in determining its severity. An irregular heart beat that has been experienced for years without any associated symptoms may be considered not critical. An irregular heart beat that increases in frequency and/ or has associated abnormal findings may be more dangerous because it limits an effective cardiac output.

## Physical Examination

### Physical Appearance

The appearance of the person with an irregular heart beat is perfectly normal unless there is an inadequate cardiac output, in which case the patient may appear ashen or clammy, be disoriented or breathless, and report light-headedness.

### Vital Signs

Dysrhythmias can be detected during measurement of the peripheral (or apical) pulses and blood pressure. An exact determination of the origin and conduction pathway of the irregular beat requires an electrocardiogram (ECG). (See Figs. 7-1 to 7-9 and diagnostic tests, below.)

#### Heart Rate

Heart rate is affected by both the demand for cardiac output and the inherent automaticity of conduction tissue. The normal sinus heart rate (NSR) is between 60 and 100 beats per minute. Both a slow heart rate (sinus bradycardia, less than 60 beats per minute) and a fast heart rate (sinus tachycardia, 100 to 160 beats per minute) are usually well tolerated under normal conditions (Fig. 7.10).

**Sinus Tachycardia.** Sinus tachycardia is a rapid but regular rate, which is normal as an exercise response. It may be seen in deconditioned patients at rest and in patients in congestive heart failure (CHF). Various drugs (e.g., methylxanthines) produce sinus tachycardia.

**Paroxysmal Atrial Tachycardia.** The pulse palpated in paroxysmal atrial tachycardia (PAT) has bursts of a very rapid rate. Figure 7.3 shows the ECG of this rapid heart rate (usually 160 to 220 beats per minute). It occurs spontaneously and is usually relieved spontaneously or with vagal nerve stimulation, including carotid massage or Valsalva maneuver. Patients

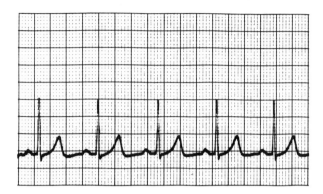

**Fig. 7.10** Normal sinus rhythm at a rate of 80 per minute. (Reproduced from Advanced Cardiac Life Support. Published by the American Heart Association, Dallas, 1983. By permission of the American Heart Association Inc.)

in generally good health can tolerate this rapid rate for several minutes. Patients with poor ventricular function or coronary artery disease (CAD) have poor tolerance to PAT owing to the shortened diastolic filling time and increased myocardial oxygen requirements to sustain this rapid rate, and such patients may experience chest pain and lightheadedness.

**Sinus Bradycardia.** Sinus bradycardia is a slow but regular rate found in very fit subjects, in persons with an increased vagal tone and myocardial ischemia, or in those receiving β blocker therapy. Bradycardia in patients with myocardial ischemia typically is associated with signs and symptoms of cardiac and/or cerebral hypoxia and is treated as a medical emergency. Figure 7.11 illustrates sinus bradycardia.

**Junctional (Nodal) Rate.** The junctional (nodal) rate is a slow rate, 40 to 60 beats per minute, with the atrioventricular (AV) node acting as the pacemaker of the heart. In subjects with good ventricular function and a normal ejection fraction, this rate can be tolerated. Because of the absence of atrial depolarization and its contribution to stroke volume (atrial "kick"), this rate may not be well tolerated in patients with ventricular dysfunction. Figure 7.12 illustrates a junctional rate in a patient with sinus node arrest.

Heart Rhythm

The palpated pulse is regular when R-R intervals on an ECG strip are equal.

An irregular rhythm can be documented by palpation of the pulse and/or by ECG. The pulse is the pressure wave created by the volume of blood that the heart has ejected. If the pulse is palpable, there has been a sufficient volume of blood delivered to the site of palpation. An irregularity in the rhythm of the pulse can be described as occurring either "regularly," with

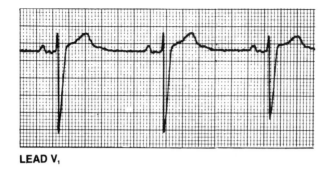

**LEAD V₁**

**Fig. 7.11** Sinus bradycardia at a rate of 46 per minute. (Reproduced from Advanced Cardiac Life Support, published by the American Heart Association, Dallas, 1983. By permission of the American Heart Association Inc.)

a consistent pattern or "irregularly," with no detectable pattern. Periods between palpable pulses are normally electrically silent; however, when the pauses are of varying time intervals, electrical depolarization and consequent contraction of some of the heart muscle may be occurring. These abnormal electrical events cause some mechanical activity of the heart muscle, but the volume of blood ejected is not sufficient to reach the periphery.

**Regularly Irregular Rhythm.** There may be no hemodynamic consequences of a dysrhythmia if the irregularity occurs infrequently (e.g., less than every six beats) and the reason for the regularly spaced prolonged intervals between beats is due to premature atrial contractions (PACs) (Table 7.1, Fig. 7.4) or premature junctional beats (PJCs) (Table 7.1, Fig. 7.5). If the prolonged intervals between perfused beats is due to premature ventricular contractions (PVCs) and these pauses are more frequent (e.g., more often than every sixth beat), lightheadedness and low blood pressure may be present (Table 7.1, Fig. 7.6).

If, for example, upon palpation of the peripheral pulse every fourth

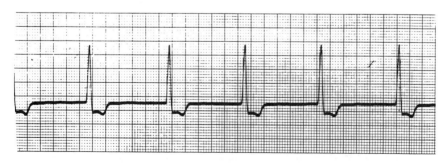

**Fig. 7.12** Junctional rate with sinus node arrest.

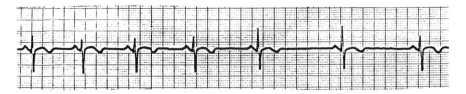

**Fig. 7.13** Sinus arrhythmia consisting of normal P-QRS-T configuration with increasing and decreasing intervals between complexes. (Reproduced from Thys D, Kaplan J: The ECG in Anesthesia and Critical Care. Churchill Livingstone, New York, 1987, with permission.)

contraction is stimulated earlier than the normal sinus paced contraction (quadragaminy), a pause will be sensed under the examiner's fingertips after three equally spaced beats have been felt. Generally, the examiner is unable to determine from peripheral palpation if the premature beat is generated from the atria or ventricles. The ECG is necessary to distinguish the source of this pause, or "skipped" beat.

Premature atrial contractions are usually well tolerated. Premature ventricular contractions are tolerated until they become frequent enough to compromise the hemodynamics and produce a low cardiac output, as is the case with ventricular tachycardia (see Fig. 9.2). The PAC is a contraction that has the benefit of some atrial volume; a PVC lacks this atrial kick and relies only on passive filling during a shortened diastole for its stroke volume. Figures 7.7 and 7.8 illustrate ECG examples of regular patterns of PVCs that are palpated as a consistently irregular rhythm. Rarely, PVCs occur before the previous beat has completed its repolarization so that the R wave of the PVC falls on the T wave of the preceding beat. This is likely to trigger ventricular tachycardia.

*Sinus Arrhythmia.* Sinus arrhythmia is a benign dysrhythmia, which is influenced by respirations, and is considered normal. It is unclear why it is more pronounced in some people and it usually normalizes during exercise. It presents as an increase in rate with inspiration and a decrease in rate with exhalation. Therefore, a consistently irregular pattern of alternating smaller and greater R–R intervals between QRS complexes on the ECG is detected. The palpable pulse feels like a regular speeding up and slowing down of the heart rate. Figure 7.13 illustrates this normal sinus arrhythmia.

**Irregularly Irregular Rhythm.** Although a patternless irregular rhythm may be a result of the erratic occurrence of PVCs or PACs, it is most commonly associated with *atrial fibrillation*. The conduction of an impulse to the ventricle is inconsistent in this dysrhythmia. There is abnormal impulse generation from the sinus node and atrial tissue so that many impulses are conducted to the AV node. There is a consequent upredictability regarding which impulse is conducted through the node to the ventricles. Figure 7.1

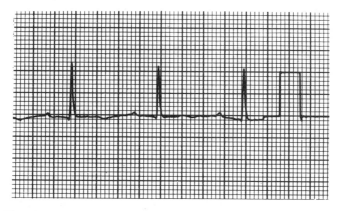

**Fig. 7.14** First-degree AV block with prolonged PR interval. (Reproduced from Thys D, Kaplan J: The ECG in Anesthesia and Critical Care. Churchill Livingstone, New York, 1987, with permission.)

illustrates atrial fibrillation, which demonstrates the absence of pattern in the RR intervals. When the atria fail to contract uniformly, the potential for blood stagnation within the atria, and particularly in the auricular appendages, is great. This facilitates clot formation and places the individual at high risk for an embolic event. Consequently, if atrial fibrillation can not be cardioverted to NSR by either pharmocologic or electrical means, then anticoagulant therapy with coumadin is usually instituted (see Ch. 4).

Patients in atrial fibrillation have a sufficient number of contractions each minute for an effective cardiac output even though the rhythm is irregular. Patients with left ventricular dysfunction, who need the atrial kick for stroke volume, may become symptomatic in atrial fibrillation.

*Atrial Flutter.*   Another atrial dysrhythmia that may consist of a patternless irregularity is atrial flutter. The ECG shows a regular atrial depolarization rate but may lack a regular ventricular response. The causes of atrial flutter are usually malignant, and this dysrhythmia is likely to deteriorate into a less organized rhythm.

*Heart Block.*   When blood supply to the AV node tissue is incomplete, delays in impulse conduction can occur. This may result in first-, second-, or third-degree AV block. In first-degree AV block, no abnormality is detected in the palpable pulse; however, the ECG does demonstrate a prolongation of the P–R interval (Fig. 7.14).

Second-degree AV block represents a more critical conduction delay in the AV node or bundle of His. At varying intervals an impulse fails to be conducted from the atria to the ventricles. At that time no pulse is palpable since there is no ventricular contraction. There are two forms of second-degree AV block:

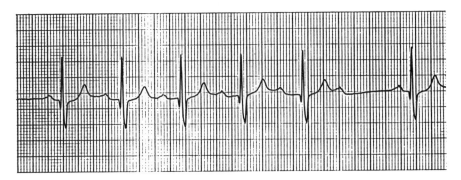

**Fig. 7.15** Second-degree AV block (Mobitz type I, Wenkebach). Note that the PR interval gradually lengthens and that the shortest PR interval follows the pause of the missing QRS complex. (Reproduced from Thys D, Kaplan J: The ECG in Anesthesia and Critical Care. Churchill Livingstone, New York, 1987, with permission.)

1. *Mobitz type I, or Wenkebach.* This form of AV block is demonstrated by a gradual prolongation of the PR interval on the ECG. Eventually a beat is dropped. This is a fairly consistent occurrence, so in fact the "pause" in the pulse may appear at regular intervals (Fig. 7.15).
2. *Mobitz type II.* This AV block causes no prolongation of the PR interval, but periodically no conduction of an atrial impulse to the ventricles follows. It is "blocked" in the AV node or bundle of His (Fig. 7.16).

In third-degree AV block (complete heart block, AV dissociation) there is no relationship between atrial depolarization and ventricular depolarization. Each occurs spontaneously at its inherent rate, and a pulse is palpated when an adequate volume of blood is ejected. A weak pulse may occur with

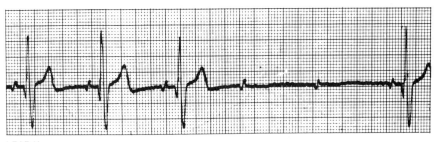

**LEAD V₂**

**Fig. 7.16** Second-degree AV block (Mobitz type II). In this example there are three conducted sinus beats followed by two nonconducted P waves. The PR interval of conducted beats remains constant. (Reproduced from Advanced Cardiac Life Support, published by American Heart Association, Dallas, 1983. By permission of the American Heart Association Inc.)

each ventricular beat if there is a large enough blood volume. Third-degree heart block is a very unstable condition, is a medical emergency, and requires a pacemaker.

*Sick Sinus Syndrome.* The pattern of heart beats in sick sinus syndrome reflects abnormal sinus node function. In this condition, in which CAD affects the sinus node blood supply either with aging or for unknown reasons, the sinus node becomes fibrotic. There are consequent and unpredictable bursts of PAT, alternating with bouts of bradycardia.

## Blood Pressure

In the presence of an irregular heart beat, blood pressure may be normal or abnormal. The closer the origin of the impulse to the SA node, the greater the stroke volume. The greater the stroke volume of each beat, the more normal the blood pressure. With a PVC stroke volume is diminished owing to the loss of atrial emptying and a blunted ventricular filling time. These factors decrease contractility by decreasing preload (Frank-Starling mechanism). The resultant drop in blood pressure activates the carotid sinus reflex to initiate peripheral vasoconstriction, which increases total peripheral resistance (TPR) and afterload to elevate the blood pressure. The normal heart responds to this increase in afterload and maintains blood pressure in spite of the PVC. In the person with left ventricular dysfunction this compensatory rise in TPR presents too great an afterload force, causing an increase in myocardial oxygen consumption and consequently overworking a left ventricle with limited reserve. Unable to further compensate, the stroke volume and blood pressure decrease, and the PVC is poorly tolerated. When the cause of the dysrhythmia is treated and stroke volume returns to normal, blood pressure normalizes as well.

## Auscultation

### Heart Sounds

Changes in the quality of the S1 and S2 can occur with an irregular heart beat. These changes are due to the alteration in blood flow and pressure created by the variable filling time between beats.

# Tests

An irregular heart beat can be due to metabolic abnormalities, causing electrolyte imbalances and/or drug toxicity, or to primary cardiac pathology, including myocardial irritability or conduction system disease. The results of the following laboratory values and tests help the physician to manage the dysrhythmia and help the therapist to understand the implications of the irregular heart beat, including its treatment and relief.

## Laboratory Values

### Potassium Levels

Elevated potassium blood levels predispose the heart muscle to electrical standstill. The cell membrane is unable to "leak" adequate sodium to enable it to depolarize. No pulse is palpable in the most extreme cases of this condition, and it is a medical emergency. Conversely, decreased blood potassium levels provoke myocardial irritability. In this condition resting membrane polarity is minimal; therefore it is easier for the cell to depolarize. The myocardial irritability primarily takes the form of ventricular ectopic activity (VEA) or PVCs. An irregular heart beat is common with decreased potassium and is rectified when potassium levels return to normal. Patients at risk of having an electrolyte disturbance (owing to diuretic therapy, dehydration, diarrhea, vomiting, or metabolic disease) routinely have potassium levels checked. See Appendix for normal potassium levels.

### Digitalis Level

Digitalis is frequently used in the treatment of CHF and atrial fibrillation. When the drug is not readily absorbed or metabolized, as in elderly patients and those with renal failure, levels may become toxic. Because digitalis also increases automaticity in secondary pacemaker tissue throughout the heart's conduction system, toxic drug levels can trigger irregular heart beats originating from variable and unpredictable foci, as in atrial fibrillation.

Normal serum digitalis levels vary with the preparation prescribed (see Appendix). Patients who are on chronic digitalis therapy and who note an increase in irregularity of their heart beat generally have their blood checked for toxic digitalis levels. (For other drug-induced cases of irregular heart beat, see section on pharmacology in this chapter.)

### Implications for Physical Therapy

Increasing irregularity of the pulse may be caused by drug toxicity, abnormal electrolytes, and myocardial ischemia. Therapists should document the finding and suggest that levels be checked.

## Electrocardiogram

The resting ECG is the single most effective way of determining the origin, the conducting pathway, and the intervals of an irregular heart beat. As described in Chapter 2, the ECG is a recording of the summation of action potentials generated from conduction tissue. Since each component of this pathway from sinoatrial node through to Purkinje fibers produces a unique waveform, the absence or predominance of a certain waveform identifies the origin of the beat. A review of all figures in this chapter demonstrate the various ECG configurations produced depending on the electrical origin

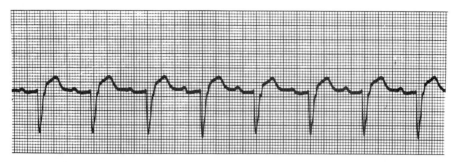

**Fig. 7.17** Bundle branch block demonstrating wide QRS complex with normal sinus rhythm.

of the beat. Numerous texts have been devoted to dysrhythmia and ECG interpretation, and the reader is encouraged to refer to those listed at the end of this chapter. Nevertheless, a few comments regarding key concepts follow.

The ECG helps to differentiate between irregularity in heart rhythm due to supraventricular and that due to ventricular impulses. In general, this distinction is valuable in anticipating the hemodynamic consequences of the irregularity. As seen in Figure 7.6, supraventricular beats have a narrow QRS complex, in contrast to those beats originating in the ventricles. The wider QRS in ventricular beats is due to slower automaticity in the Purkinje fibers. It should also be noted that conduction delays in the bundle branches can cause a widening of the QRS complex as well. These beats generate a regular pulse, and each beat is associated with atrial depolarization in NSR. See Figure 7.17.

### Exercise Tolerance Test

As noted in previous chapters, the resting ECG is valuable if a symptom is present all the time. Often, however, an irregular heart beat only occurs during a high catecholamine state or when there is an imbalance between myocardial oxygen supply and demand. The controlled setting provided during an exercise tolerance test (ETT) not only allows the safe provocation and detection of the originating focus of certain irregular heart beats but also determines the functional consequences of the irregularity. Conservative reports estimate that 25 percent of the normal population exhibit VEA with exercise without hemodynamic impairment or resultant lightheadedness or drop in blood pressure.[1] As stated previously, the more frequent the ectopy, the greater the risk of hemodynamic compromise. Figure 7.18 illustrates the onset of T wave inversion, ST segment depression, and a PVC with increasing work during an ETT. (For more information on ETT see Ch. 4.)

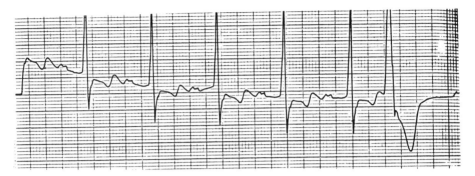

**Fig. 7.18** Onset of ST segment and T wave changes and PVCs with exercise. (Feinberg, B: Preoperative Diagnosis of Myocardial Ischemia. p. 103. In Thys DM, Kaplan JA (eds): The ECG in Anesthesia and Critical Care. Churchill Livingstone, New York, 1987 with permission.)

## Holter Monitor

The Holter monitor is an ambulatory ECG monitoring device. Its primary use is for dysrhythmia detection and documentation. Chest electrodes are placed on the patient and are attached to a portable tape recorder for a set period of time, typically 8 or 24 hours. The patient is instructed to carry out normal daily activities and to maintain a written log of activities and any symptoms. In this way, dysrhythmias appearing on the tape can be correlated with symptoms to help the physician interpret the functional significance of the abnormality (see Ch. 4.)

## Electrophysiologic Studies

Electrophysiologic studies (EPS) involve the percutaneous insertion of several multipolar catheters, predominantly into the right side of the heart. This is usually done via the femoral vein under local anesthesia. These electrode catheters allow two types of studies to be performed.[2]

The first evaluation involves the passive recording of the electrical potential at different sites in the heart. This is useful in evaluating heart blocks and the need for and type of permanent pacemaker. This type of recording offers little or no discomfort to the patient and there are minimal risks associated with the procedure.

The second kind of evaluation possible during an EPS is to determine the morphology and clinical significance of potentially lethal dysrhythmias when they are not caused by ischemia. The test involves a series of electrical stimulations delivered to the myocardium to induce the clinical dysrhythmia being investigated. There is a twofold benefit to dysrhythmia induction in this clinical setting. First, if signs and symptoms of hemodynamic compromise are associated with the dysrhythmia, immediate intervention can be made. Second, the appropriate drugs to be used in treatment of the conduction disturbance can be determined. Frequently this requires repeat testing, initially to determine the stimulus required to induce the dysrhythmia and subsequently to try to provoke the dysrhythmia after an antiarrhythmic agent has been prescribed. Multiple sequences of drug loading followed by EPS may be required to determine a drug and dosage that are both suitable to inhibit the dysrhythmia and that will have minimal side effects on the patient.

It is important to realize that when the dysrhythmia is provoked, it frequently causes a hemodynamically significant response, and electrical defibrillation is often required to correct the conduction disturbance. Needless to say, this can become extremely traumatic to a patient.

As a result of EPS testing recommendations can be made for dysrhythmia suppression by means other than drug therapy. These include ablation therapy, overdrive pacemakers, surgical resection of the cells generating the ectopic focus, or use of an automatic implantable defibrillator (AID).

Implications for Physical Therapy

Patients can benefit from an endurance program as long as (1) the tests verify that dysrhythmia is not due to ischemia and (2) an antiarrhythmic agent is being taken so that the probability of a dysrhythmic event occurring is no greater with exercise than at rest.

Patients may have a new drug for dysrhythmia control following an EPS. Therapists should recognize new symptoms that occur from changes in drugs.

If a new drug has not reached therapeutic range, exercise should be closely monitored.

Patients who have experienced multiple defibrillations may need extra emotional support.

## MEDICAL-SURGICAL INTERVENTION

# Pharmacology

When the origin and mechanism of conduction of the irregular heart beat is known, the appropriate drug can be prescribed. The pharmocologic treatment of diseases causing ectopy, such as CAD or pulmonary disease, is discussed in Chapters 4 and 5.

### Antiarrhythmics

Antiarrhythmic drugs are used primarily for the control of ventricular dysrhythmias or supraventricular tachycardia. Although any conduction tissue cell has the capacity to generate an impulse (automaticity), normally the sinus node establishes the pace of myocardial depolarization. Other conduction tissue produces the impulse if sinus node stimulus production fails, if myocardial tissue becomes ischemic with excessive irritability, or if depolarization of the ventricles is not synchronous. Recall that there is a protective mechanism in the event of a failure of the SA node to initiate the impulse, which entails spontaneous firing of distal conduction tissue at a slower rate (see Ch. 2).

Treatment to correct this compensatory slow rate is not usually undertaken unless the cardiac output is compromised and/or symptoms occur. However, when the cause of a dysrhythmia is not due to the protective "escape" mechanism of conduction tissue, increased automaticity and re-entry causes most irregular heart beats. Figure 7.19 illustrates the re-entry mechanism of dysrhythmia production.

Cells that are ischemic may take longer than most other cells to conduct the impulse (i.e., to depolarize) and repolarize. As demonstrated in Figure 7.19, by the time ischemic muscle depolarizes, adjacent healthy muscle tissue may already have repolarized and can respond to this impulse, which reaches it before the new normal impulse from the SA node. Hence, there is a new impulse originating from an ectopic focus in the ventricles, or a PVC on the ECG.

Pharmacologic intervention can either: (1) improve conduction through the ischemic zone so that the normal impulse can proceed forward fast enough for cells to be refractory to an impulse arriving from neighboring tissue; or (2) decrease impulse conduction through the ischemic zone so that impulses arriving from neighboring tissue in a retrograde fashion cannot be conducted.

Antiarrhythmic drugs are classified according to action. The four classes of medications, their indications, and side effects are found in Table 7.2.

## Digitalis

Digitalis is primarily used for its inotropic properties in heart failure. It is also used for the management of dysrhythmias, particularly those originating in the atria. Digitalis has the following electrophysiologic effects: (1) increases automaticity of secondary pacemakers in the heart (atria, AV node, bundle of His, Purkinje fibers); (2) decreases impulse conduction in the heart; (3) increases refractory period of specialized conduction cells and myocardial cells. Unfortunately, as discussed previously in this chapter, digitalis toxicity is common and causes a variety of dysrhythmias, including PVCs (bigeminy, multifocal), ventricular tachycardia, first-, second-, and third-degree AV block, atrial fibrillation, PAT with block, PACs, atrial flutter, sinus tachycardia, sinus bradycardia, sinus arrest, nodal tachycardia, nodal rhythm, and nodal premature beats.[1]

Digitalis is often the drug of choice in the treatment of superventricular dysrhythmias associated with an acute myocardial infarction (see Table 4.8).

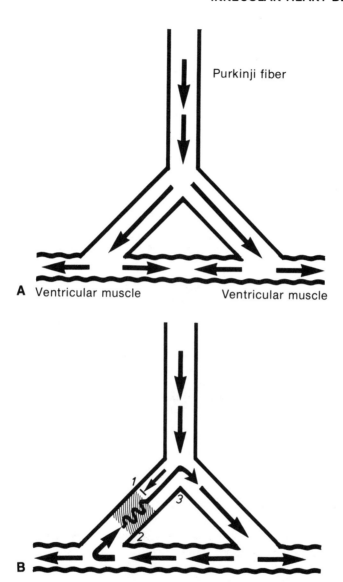

**Fig. 7.19** (**A**) Normal conduction pathway of a depolarization wave through a Purkinje fiber to ventricular muscle. The depolarization wave arrives simultaneously at all portions of ventricular muscle and then extinguishes. (**B**) Re-entry circuit model with unidirectional block. The depolarization wave is blocked at the ischemic zone (1); however, it is able to depolarize the ventricular muscle from the opposite direction (2). By the time the impulse passes through this ischemic area, the healthy muscle is repolarized and responds to this impulse (3) before the next impulse can be generated from the SA node. (Modified from Tyndall A: A nursing perspective of the invasive approach to treatment of ventricular arrhythmias. Heart Lung 12:6, 1983.)

Table 7.2 **Indications and Side Effects of Commonly Used Antiarryhthymic Drugs**

| Class | Drug | Indications | Side Effects |
|---|---|---|---|
| I[a] | Quinidine | Paroxysmal supraventricular tachycardia; atrial fibrillation; atrial flutter; PVCs; ventricular tachycardia; digitalis toxicity | GI, thrombocytopenia, rash |
| | Procainamide | | GI, thrombocytopenia, lupus syndrome |
| | Disopyramide | | Urinary obstruction |
| | Lidocaine | | CNS, confusion, seizure |
| | Tocainide | | GI, CNS, dizzy, vertigo, paresthesia, rash |
| | Phenytoin | | Hypotension, respiratory arrest |
| II | Propranolol | Paroxysmal supraventricular tachycardia; Atrial fibrillation; PVCs; Ventricular tachycardia | Decreased HR; Decreased inotropy; Bronchospasm |
| III | Bretylium tosylate | Ventricular tachycardia; Ventricular fibrillation | Postural hypotension; Occasionally sinus tachycardia |
| | Amiodarone hydrochloride | Atrial and ventricular dysrhythmias | Corneal micro deposits; Tremors; Insomnia; Ataxia; Proximal muscle weakness |
| IV | Verapamil | Paroxysmal supraventricular tachycardia; Atrial fibrillation | Hypotension; Headache |

[a] Indications for all Class I drugs are the same.
(Adapted from Ice D: Cardiovascular Medications. Phys Ther 65(12):56, 1985.)

## Rehabilitation

The therapeutic benefits of a comprehensive rehabilitation program for patients with an irregular heart beat have not been systematically studied. Atrial dysrhythmias are usually well tolerated at rest and during exercise as long as they do not increase in frequency or compromise cardiac output. If the underlying cause of the atrial dysrhythmia is known and is stable, these patients can benefit from a program of behavior modification to promote health and wellness and CAD prevention. An aerobic training program will benefit patients who have atrial dysrhythmias by improving oxygen transport capabilities. There is no evidence showing that training will alter the dysrhythmia.

Atrial fibrillation is not usually a life-threatening dysrhythmia. In fact, some people remain in this rhythm for much of their elderly adult lives. A new onset of atrial fibrillation may indicate serious cardiac pathology and requires early medical attention.

Patients with atrial fibrillation should be exercise-tested to obtain a training heart rate range by observing the changes in ventricular response rate with exercise. This increases with greater work loads, and the radial pulse may feel more regular as the heart rate response speeds up.

Patients with an irregular heart beat due to ventricular dysrhythmias may well benefit from the emotional, educational, and exercise components of a formal rehabilitation program. The rehabilitation process for patients with ischemia-induced VEA is addressed in Chapter 4. The following section focuses on the possible benefits of a rehabilitation program for patients with primary ventricular conduction abnormalities.

### Emotional and Educational Support

In this discussion two areas will be addressed. First, patients with significant VEA may be very frightened. They may have personal knowledge of sudden death without any apparent provocation. Subsequent diagnostic tests, including EPS, may have induced the dysrhythmia and required electrical cardioversion, causing further anxiety. Patients may feel as if they are "walking time bombs." Support groups and the opportunity to discuss their feelings with health care providers can be very helpful. Explanations regarding the effectiveness of a patient's drug regimen can be reassuring. Teaching patients how to take their own pulse and monitor its rhythm allows them to detect increases in VEA before it becomes significant.

The second area of major concern deals with the hypothesis that overstimulation of the sympathetic nervous system from emotional stress may influence electrophysiologic properties of the myocardium and consequently aggravate or even precipitate dysrhythmias.[3] When patients who have experienced VEA and/or sudden death are faced with stressful tasks, the frequency of ventricular ectopy has been shown to increase.[4] Patients report an increase in their irregular heart beat during periods of significant change in their lives, such as divorce, grief, or altered work patterns. Although health care providers cannot alter a life crisis, patients can benefit from support and guidance in responding to unusual stresses in a healthy manner. There is evidence that patients who sincerely believe in the effectiveness of their therapeutic program show a reduction in VEA.[5]

### Exercise Program

Exercise intervention has not been a major therapeutic modality used in the treatment of patients with recurrent VEA. There are two indications for using exercise therapy with this population when the dysrhythmia is unrelated to myocardial ischemia and CAD.

Patients undergoing EPS for evaluation of the efficacy of drug therapies may be hospitalized for prolonged periods of time. They may benefit from stationary bicycling and other forms of aerobic activity to prevent them from deconditioning. Their ectopy is usually unrelated to exertion, and the positive psychological effects of exercise may even reduce the frequency of dysrhythmia production. These patients are closely monitored during ex-

Table 7.3 Standard Pacemaker Codes

| Chamber(s) Paced | Chamber(s) Sensed | Mode of Response |
|---|---|---|
| V = ventricle | V = ventricle | T = triggered |
| A = atria | A = atria | I = inhibited |
| D = both A and V | D = both A and V | D = both T and I |
| | O = no sensing | O = no response |

(Reproduced from Levine P, Mace R: Pacing Therapy: A Guide to Cardiac Pacing for Optimum Hemodynamic Benefit. p. 65. Futura Publishing Co., Mt. Kisco, NY 1983.)

ercise. A defibrillator and personnel trained in its use should always be nearby.

There have been some very preliminary data from South Africa showing that exercise training in rats increased the myocardial resistance to electrically induced ventricular fibrillation.[6] Although this experimental model cannot be applied to man directly, the results of the study may support epidemiologic studies reporting lower death rates among physically active men and women.[7]

## Invasive Monitoring

See electrophysiologic studies in this chapter.

## Invasive Procedures

### Pacemaker

Pacemakers are devices that stimulate cardiac muscle contraction and thereby produce an effective cardiac output in the case of a conduction deficit. When an irregular heart beat is caused by a block in conduction (second- or third-degree AV block), a permanent pacemaker may be indicated. Similarly, if automaticity of the sinus node fails (sinus arrest) and junctional or ventricular "escape" beats "pace" the heart slowly and unpredictably, pacemaker therapy may be required.

Pacemaker technology has become increasingly complex. Early devices, which set the heart rate at a "fixed" frequency irrespective of the natural sinus node pace, are rarely used. Most units currently in use act on demand and sense the occurrence of intrinsic cardiac activity. They respond to this activity either by inhibiting the pacemaker output (I) or by triggering it (T). The inhibiting mode is more common.

Whenever a pacemaker "fires" an impulse, a narrow spike appears on the ECG. This pacing spike may fall in the middle of or before the P wave if the electrode is in the atrium, or in or before the QRS complex if the electrode is in the ventricle. If a spike appears on the ECG but an appropriate P wave or QRS complex fails to be produced, the pacemaker failed to "capture" or achieve a stimulation threshold.

In order to more easily identify pacemaker function, a standard three-letter code system is employed (see Table 7.3).[8]

When both chambers are paced, the intent is to augment stroke volume by proper coordination of atrial and ventricular systole. Recent advances in dual-chamber pacing have been of great value for patients with left ventricular dysfunction. Factors besides ventricular function that are involved in the determination of the kind of pacemaker used include the type of conduction deficit and a patient's age and life-style.

Pacemakers may be placed temporarily or permanently. Both types consist of a pacing electrode and a power source. An electrode catheter is directed transvenously to the right side of the heart, and the tip is anchored into the trabeculae of the auricle or ventricle. The electrode wire is connected to the power source, which for the permanent pacemaker is typically implanted in the right infraclavicular fossa. When a device is used temporarily, the transvenous wires are attached to an external power source at the right subclavian or antecubital vein. Vigorous movements in the first 24 to 48 hours after implantation of a permanent pacemaker can displace the electrode or possibly break the wire. Either of these problems may cause the pacemaker to fail to sense or capture appropriately. This may produce an irregular heart beat, with or without hemodynamic consequences. Another cause of pacemaker malfunction is an aging battery.

### Aneurysmectomy/Myectomy

Occasionally, an area of functional but ischemic heart muscle remains bordering an infarcted or aneurysmal region. The ischemic area has a lower threshold of automaticity and often causes ventricular dysrhythmias, including ventricular tachycardia and fibrillation. Surgical excision of the myocardial tissue containing the ectopic focus (myectomy) is an alternative treatment for a hemodynamically significant dysrhythmia when more conservative medical therapy is ineffective. Dilated and globally hypokinetic ventricles do not repond to this surgery as well as those with discrete irritable foci.

### Ablation Therapy

Ablation therapy is in its early development and is considered experimental. It is primarily reserved for patients who are at too great risk for major surgery but who have ventricular dysrhythmias that are potentially lethal or of functional significance and are refractory to medical management.

In this technique a catheter is introduced into the heart chamber and directed to the region of myocardium exhibiting increased automaticity (as determined previously by EPS). The area of muscle is actually killed, or ablated, to render the tissue electrically silent. The amount of muscle damage is typically minimal, with no significant compromise of ventricular function.

An increase in cardiac enzymes consistent with myocardial necrosis does occur.

### Automatic Implantable Defibrillator

The AID is used in very select patients who exhibit repeated ventricular tachycardia or ventricular fibrillation that is not well controlled by medication. The device consists of two electrodes and a power source. The power source, which is implanted in the patient's abdomen subcutaneously, detects a dysrhythmia and delivers an electrical shock across the myocardium to return the heart to normal sinus rhythm. There is no limit to the number of shocks it can deliver as long as the power source is functional. Additional investigations of the effectiveness and usefulness of the AID will be necessary before it becomes more widely available.[9]

## PHYSICAL THERAPY INTERVENTION

## Interview

Patients exhibiting an irregular heart beat or having a history of dysrhythmia are frequently on medications to control it. They may not be able to associate any symptoms with the irregularity; however, certain key questions should be asked during the interview. Add the following key questions to the generic physical therapy patient interview:

1. Describe the sensation.
2. Under what conditions do you get this sensation?
3. What do you do when you experience this sensation?
4. What do you think is causing your irregular heart beat?
5. Do you have any special thoughts when this sensation occurs?

## Evaluation

### Musculoskeletal Evaluation

See Chapter 3.

### Cardiopulmonary Evaluation

Abnormal findings from the cardiopulmonary evaluation (see Ch. 3) reflect the hemodynamic dysfunction caused by the dysrhythmia. When symptoms are produced by a dysrhythmia, further cardiopulmonary evaluation should be made (see Chapters 4, 5, and 8 for specific procedures) to establish the functional significance of the dysrhythmia. Alterations in heart rate, rhythm, blood pressure, and ECG are important components of the evaluation of an irregular heart beat.

Vital Signs

**Heart Rate.** In the presence of an irregular heart beat, the heart rate is counted for a full minute to determine the total number of fully perfused beats.

**Heart Rhythm.** The heart rhythm is evaluated both peripherally and apically. The peripheral pulse is described as regular, regularly irregular, or irregularly irregular. When regular pauses are noted in the peripheral pulse, apical auscultation can be simultaneously performed. The presence or absence of a heart sound during a pause is noted. Any findings associated with the time of the pause, or skipped beat (such as a palpitation, heart flipflop, or flutter) are recorded, as is the frequency with which the pause occurs each minute.

**Blood Pressure.** Care is taken during the measurement of blood pressure when there is an irregular heart beat. Pauses can be heard during cuff deflation. The examiner may overestimate diastolic pressure, mistaking the absence of a timely next beat for cessation of sound. The prolonged interval before the next sinus beat may be due to an ectopic beat.

Electrocardiogram

The resting rhythm strip of a single ECG lead helps to identify the irregular beat. Consecutive beats are checked for the presence of a complete P-QRS-T complex occurring at regular intervals. Segments of this waveform may be prolonged, missing, or dissociated in heart block or sinus arrest and can account for an irregular heart beat. Next, the onset of any premature beat with regard to the previous beat is noted. Premature beats may occur very early after a previous beat or may occur just before their normal time. The frequency of the abnormal pattern (bigeminy for every second beat or trigeminy for every third) is documented. In addition, the configuration of premature beats is described, whether they are wide or narrow, uniform (originating from a single ectopic focus) or multiform (originating from several ectopic foci). The absence or presence of additional symptoms simultaneous with dysrhythmia detection on the rhythm strip is documented and further evaluated.

## Functional Evaluation

The significance of an irregular heart beat can be determined from a functional evaluation. Activity causes an increase in myocardial work, which in turn can stimulate the abnormality when its onset is related to increased myocardial demand.

A patient should be instructed to perform various routine tasks pertinent to the physical therapy exercise program, during which the therapist monitors heart rate, heart rhythm, blood pressure, and ECG rhythm strip. All changes in these variables from resting values are documented. Particular attention is given to recognizing the following changes as work progresses: (1) increases or decreases in frequency of dysrhythmias; (2) alterations in origin of dysrhythmias; (3) development of new foci; (4) blood pressure responses when the dysrhythmia occurs; (5) any sensations such as palpitations or flutter that are associated with the dysrhythmia; (6) any symptoms such as lightheadedness, chest pain, breathlessness, confusion, or pallor that are associated with the dysrhythmia; and (7) time taken to return to resting values when work stops.

Any exercise or activity program should not exceed an intensity that provokes ventricular irritability or hemodynamic compromise. An aerobic conditioning program can be prescribed following the guidelines found in Chapter 4. Instruction and practice in relaxation techniques may offer some help in reducing the occurrence of VEA and should be included in a comprehensive therapy program.

## REFERENCES

1. Sokolow M, McIlroy M: Clinical Cardiology. Lange Medical Books, Los Altos, CA, 1981
2. Haffagee C: When to do cardiac electrophysiologic studies. (Abstr) New England Cardiovascular Society, Symp. on "Recent Advances in Cardiovascular Diseases, 1987. American Heart Association, Massachussetts Affiliate, 1987
3. Lown B: Clinical management of ventricular arryhthmias. Hosp Prac, 73, Apr 1982
4. Ornish D: Stress, Diet, and Your Heart. New American Library, New York, 1982
5. Benson H: Beyond the Relaxation Response. Times Books, New York, 1984
6. Noakes T, Higginson L, Opie L: Physical training increases ventricular fibrillation thresholds of isolated rat hearts during normoxia, hypoxia, and regional ischemia. Circulation 67(1):24, 1983
7. Paffenbarger R, Hyde ZR, Wing Y: Physical activity, all-cause mortality, and longevity of college alumni. N Engl J Med 314:605, 1986
8. Levine P, Mace R: Pacing Therapy: A Guide to Cardiac Pacing for Optimum Hemodynamic Benefit. Futura Publishing Co., New York, 1983
9. Mirowski M, Reid P, Winkle R, et al: "Reduction in predicted mortality from malignant ventricular arrhythmias following implantation of the automatic defibrillator. J Am Coll Card 1:609, 1983

## SUGGESTED READINGS

McIntyre K, Lewis J (eds): Textbook of Advanced Cardiac Life Support. American Heart Association, 1983
Dubin D: Rapid ECG Interpretation. 3rd Ed., Cover Publishing Co., Tampa, FL, 1974

Ellestad M: Stress Testing. Principles and Practice. 2nd Ed., FA Davis, Philadelphia, 1980

Netter F: The Ciba Collection of Medical Illustrations. The Heart. Vol. 5, Ciba-Geigy, West Caldwell, NJ, 1969

Tyndall A: A nursing perspective of the invasive approach to treatment of ventricular arrhythmias. Heart Lung 12:621, 1983

# LIGHTHEADEDNESS 8

The patient who complains of lightheadedness or dizziness may be seriously ill, with decreased oxygen being delivered to the brain. Conversely, this symptom may reflect a typical cold or influenza. Therefore, immediate information regarding associated symptoms should be sought when lightheadedness is present. Examples of the more serious causes of lightheadedness are found in the Table 8.1 and will be discussed in this chapter.

## CHART REVIEW

### Medical History

A review of the medical history is made to recognize the setting in which the symptom occurs and its sequelae. Patients with known dysrhythmias, orthostasis, hypotension, poor ventricular function, diabetes mellitus, and coronary artery disease (CAD) are at high risk for experiencing lightheadedness. High anxiety and emotional stress can cause hyperventilation, which will produce lightheadedness. Anxiety alone can stimulate vagal discharge and produce lightheadedness. Occasionally, lightheadedness may reflect an intolerance to different drugs or doses. Knowledge of these confounding factors adds insight in understanding and managing lightheadedness.

In a patient with new onset of lightheadedness, information regarding activities the patient was doing at the time the symptom was experienced is essential. A quick change in a prolonged position, physical exertion such as lifting, pushing, or straining with a bowel movement will reduce venous return, potentially dropping the blood pressure, which can result in lightheadedness. Patients with aortic stenosis are more likely to experience lightheadedness with these maneuvers.

It is important to ascertain from the medical history how long the symptom lasts, how often it occurs, how it is relieved, and whether it leads to loss of consciousness. Lightheadedness associated with coronary insufficiency may not be relieved until the myocardial oxygen demand is decreased

**171**

**Table 8.1 Differential Diagnosis of Lightheadedness**

| Possible Causes | Possible Findings | Stimuli | Pathology |
|---|---|---|---|
| Ventricular ectopic activity | Irregular heart beat; low blood pressure; pallor; "palpitations"; can lead to loss of consciousness | Low potassium<br>Caffeine<br>Any hypermetabolic state<br>Myocardial or cerebral ischemia | Myocardial dysfunction<br>Acute cerebrovascular accident |
| Hypotension | Low blood pressure; low pulse pressure; loss of consciousness; increased heart rate; pallor | Valsalva<br>Drugs<br>Orthostatic intolerance<br>Hypovolemia | Peripheral vasodilation<br>Cardiogenic shock |
| Cerebral ischemia | Slurred speech; hemiparesis; blurred vision; incoordination; headache; disorientation | Trauma<br>Brain hypoxia<br>Carotid artery lesion<br>Cerebral artery aneurysm | Cerebral atherosclerosis<br>Cerebrovascular accident |
| Vasovagal syncope | Decreased blood pressure; decreased heart rate; pallor; tinnitus; diaphoresis, rapid recovery in supine position | Fear (e.g., at sight of blood)<br>High anxiety state | Vagal stimulation |
| Hyperventilation | Increased respiratory rate; pallor; diaphoresis; decreased $PCO_2$ | Fear<br>High anxiety state<br>Hypercarbia<br>Hypoxia | Respiratory or metabolic acidosis |
| Hypoglycemia | Diaphoresis; ketone breath; confusion; fatigue, pallor | Exercise<br>Decreased food intake<br>Inappropriate insulin | Diabetes mellitus |

or coronary blood supply is increased. Methods of relief may include rest, medication, or emergency medical intervention (see Ch. 4).

Does oral administration of a fast-acting carbohydrate (orange juice, hard candy) relieve the symptom in the diabetic? Does water ingestion reverse the lightheadedness caused by hypovolemia? Has carotid massage, drugs, and/or electrical cardioversion been necessary to return the patient to normal sinus rhythm? In the case of a sustained supraventricular tachycardia or paroxysmal atrial fibrillation, medical attention may be necessary to reverse the symptom. If lightheadedness progresses to loss of consciousness, a life-threatening emergency may exist as in the case of ventricular tachycardia and fibrillation or complete heart block and asystole (see Ch. 9).

### Implications for Physical Therapy

If the patient has ventricular ectopic activity (VEA) or an irregular pulse, the therapist should monitor the patient with a rhythm strip (ECG).

If the patient is diabetic, have a quick acting carbohydrate source available.

Be sure that emergency medical backup is available.

Check that the patient is well hydrated.

## Physical Examination

### Physical Appearance

Patients with lightheadedness may look pale and be sweaty and limp. If patients rapidly lose consciousness, they will either recover quickly in recumbency or there is reason to initiate cardiopulmonary resuscitation. Diabetics who lose consciousness require an injection of glucagon to increase their blood glucose. If there is cerebral ischemia associated with lightheadedness, the patient may exhibit a hemiparesis, incoordination, and slurred speech.

### Vital Signs

#### Heart Rate

The heart rate may be very fast or unusually slow in the alert patient with lightheadedness. A sinus tachycardia (100 to 160 beats per minute) or paroxysmal atrial tachycardia (160 to 220 beats per minute) means that the heart is beating too fast to allow effective filling of the ventricle because of a shortened diastolic phase. In these cases blood pressure decreases owing to the decreased preload and causes lightheadedness. In sinus bradycardia (less than 60 beats per minute) or a junctional (40 to 60 beats per minute) or ventricular rhythm (less than 40 beats per minute), the cardiac output may be inadequate for cerebral perfusion. The patient may remain conscious owing to a very effective stroke volume and low peripheral demand. Lightheadedness may also be the case when an external demand pacemaker fails to function.

### Heart Rhythm

Determination of the regularity of the pulse is essential in the management of the patient with lightheadedness. If a patient with a known irregularity of the heart rhythm is symptomatic, this may or may not be due to the abnormal rhythm, and much more documentation is necessary. The patient with a new onset of an irregular heart beat will most likely be symptomatic because of a decreased cardiac output. The irregularity in the heart rhythm indicates alterations in impulse conduction, which may compromise stroke volume, triggering lightheadedness (see Ch. 7).

### Blood Pressure

A drop in blood pressure typically results in the symptom of lightheadedness due to decreased oxygen delivery to the brain. A primary drop in blood pressure occurs when there is significant peripheral vasodilation. Reduction in vasomotor tone is induced by agents such as nitrates, captopril, or prazosin (see Tables 4.6 and 4.7) and by fear and tremendous stress. Bleeding or other loss of blood volume, as in dehydration due to diaphoresis or excessive diuresis, can cause lightheadedness due to preload reduction. In these instances the symptom is usually relieved by a supine position, administration of fluids, and occasionally medications to induce vasoconstriction.

When a drop in blood pressure is caused by an irregular heart beat, a tachycardia, or a bradycardia, adjustment of the heart rate and rhythm typically returns the blood pressure to normal and reverses lightheadedness. In instances in which primary myocardial disease is present, as in CAD, valvular disease or cardiomyopathy, surgical or medical treatment of the problem can help relieve lightheadedness due to low blood pressure and its associated symptoms.

### Respiratory Rate

When the respiratory rate rises in excess of the metabolic requirement to eliminate $CO_2$, too much $CO_2$ is blown off, the $PCO_2$ falls, and the pH rises, producing a respiratory alkalosis. Lightheadedness is experienced because the hemoglobin affinity for $O_2$ is higher and its release to the tissues is made more difficult. The brain receives less $O_2$ than it requires, and lightheadedness is the first symptom of this.

### Temperature

An elevated core temperature results in tachycardia and could provoke a dysrhythmia, producing lightheadedness (see Ch. 7.)

# Tests

## Laboratory Values

There are a few instances in which chemical imbalances in the body cause lightheadedness. Some of these are discussed below.

### Potassium Level

When potassium levels in the serum are decreased myocardial cellular membrane potential is closer to zero. The cells remain more easily depolarized and are therefore in a more irritable state. In such cases there is a greater likelihood of ventricular ectopy occurring. This can cause lightheadedness due to a decreased stroke volume. Decreased potassium levels are found in patients who have lost electrolytes from vomiting or diarrhea or from potent diuretic therapy. The latter includes use of hydrochlorothiazide, Lasix, and other diuretics (see Tables 4.6 and 4.7). Normal serum potassium is 3.5 to 5.2 mEq/L (see Ch. 4).

### Digitalis Level

The primary use of digitalis is to increase contractility in heart failure. It also decreases atrioventricular conduction and slows the ventricular rate when atrial fibrillation is present. At toxic levels digitalis has potent electrophysiologic effects, which may result in lightheadedness. Effects include exacerbation of ectopic, atrial, or ventricular rhythms due to increased automaticity of pacemaker tissue. Older patients or those with impaired renal function may not absorb and metabolize digitalis efficiently and easily become toxic. Normal serum levels of digoxin and digitoxin are 0.5 to 2.5 and 20 to 35 ng/ml, respectively. (See Ch. 7.)

### Glucose Level

Cell function is dependent on the presence of blood glucose. When blood levels are inadequate for metabolic processes, a patient may complain of lightheadedness. Insulin, produced by the pancreas, regulates glucose utilization. Patients with diabetes mellitus have a defective glucose regulatory system; they may produce inadequate amounts of insulin or may exhibit insulin resistance. Exogenous insulin or oral diabetic agents (sulfonylureas) enable glucose to be utilized in these patients. Effective management of the patient with diabetes requires an adequate balance of three factors: food or caloric intake, exercise or caloric expense, and insulin. A change in one or more of these factors usually requires a change in another factor. For example, a decrease in food intake without a decrease in exercise or decrease in insulin can leave the patient relatively hypoglycemic and feeling lightheaded and weak. Quick administration of substances high in sugar raises blood glucose levels and relieves the patient's symptoms. During vigorous exercise glucose is metabolized for energy at a faster rate than usual. In such cases patients with diabetes mellitus who administer their usual insulin dose will likely become hypoglycemic with symptoms unless food intake is increased. Therefore, diabetic patients who participate in aerobic exercise require less insulin since the exercise demands facilitate glucose utilization. In addition insulin uptake and glucose utilization are facilitated in the intramuscular injection site if the injected muscle is actively exercised. Therefore, in order to avoid a hypoglycemic reaction patients should be instructed to inject insulin into a less active muscle group (only one solution to the problem).

In the fasting subject blood glucose should be 80 to 120 mg per 100 ml. Higher levels may reflect diabetes mellitus. Noninsulin dependent diabetics (NIDDM) can effectively monitor their own glucose level by testing glucose spillage in the urine; however a negative urine test may be misleading. The renal threshold for glucose to appear in the urine may be a blood glucose as high as 300 mg/dl. Many diabetologists are currently asking patients to do self-monitored blood glucose tests (SMBG). This involves sampling blood by finger prick several times a day and adjusting the insulin dose accordingly. In any 24-hour period the variability in blood glucose is a consequence of changes in metabolic need created by exercise, diet, emotional and physical stress, and intercurrent illness.[1] Hence in order to keep the diabetic as normoglycemic as possible, frequent blood testing is recommended.

## Hemoglobin A1c

A certain amount of glucose normally is irreversibly linked to hemoglobin; this is called *glycosylated hemoglobin, glycohemoglobin,* or hemoglobin A1c. When HbA1c is measured in the blood of an intensively well controlled diabetic, its concentration may be close to the normal range (3 to 6 percent) because it represents average blood glucose over time. Changes in the blood glucose level in either direction in the preceding 5 to 6 weeks will be reflected in present HbA1c blood levels. With prolonged hyperglycemia, levels of HbA1c may rise as high as 18 to 20 percent. After normoglycemic levels are stabilized, HbA1c levels return to normal in about 3 weeks.[1]

## Miscellaneous Laboratory Tests

Certain diseases (blood neoplasms and sickle cell anemia or other genetic deficiency diseases) or drugs (cytotoxin, methyldopa, quinidine) can cause anemia, which can induce lightheadedness. Hemoglobin and hematocrit values reflect the oxygen-carrying capacity of the blood and when low can cause this symptom. It should be noted that although each isolated condition may not cause lightheadedness, when mild forms of these conditions are in combination with other cardiovascular pathology, lightheadedness may be induced.

**Implications for Physical Therapy**
1. Check relevant laboratory values for level, and make sure value is *recent.*
2. Suggest repeat test if necessary.

## Electrocardiogram

Pertinent findings in the medical record regarding the 12-lead ECG or rhythm strip can add insight into the cause of a patient's complaint of lightheadedness. In the case of an irregular rhythm, either regularly or irregularly irregular, the ECG shows the origin of the impulse and its conduction. If the impulse originates in the sinus node but is not consistently conducted through the ventricles, delivery of an inadequate blood volume to the brain may cause lightheadedness. This is due to a nonsequential depolarization of cardiac chambers, which stimulates a nonsequential contraction. Similarly, if the origin of the impulse is below the sinoatrial node, the contraction that follows this stimulus is incomplete, ejecting only partial contents of the cardiac chambers; this can cause lightheadedness due to the inadequate blood volume pumped to the brain.

The frequency with which these abnormal impulses occur affects the patient's tolerance to them. An occasional "ectopic" beat should not compromise a healthy heart. When there is a contractile deficit, as with a previous myocardial infarction or cardiomyopathy, even one ectopic beat can compromise the cardiac output.

Rhythm abnormalities associated with symptoms caused by low tissue perfusion are routinely treated. An ECG is used to monitor the success of treatments such as pacemaker therapy, antiarrhythmic medication, and cardioversion (see Ch. 7).

## Exercise Tolerance Test

In cases in which angina is atypical and coronary underperfusion presents as lightheadedness, the exercise test can confirm the diagnosis of myocardial ischemia. The exercise ECG can help determine whether lightheadedness is a symptom of myocardial ischemia, as verified by ECG changes or by radioisotope perfusion abnormalities. Lightheadedness caused by ventricular ectopy or inotropic incompetence can be reproduced by the stress of exercise. In such cases medical therapy is directed toward reducing myocardial irritability or optimizing ventricular function. This may include pharmacologic, rehabilitative, or invasive interventions (see Chs. 4 and 7).

## Implication for Physical Therapy

If VEA is induced by exercise, monitor ECG during physical therapy exercise and keep exercise intensity lower than threshold of lightheadedness.

## Holter Monitor

The Holter monitor is a form of ambulatory ECG monitoring and is typically applied for 8 to 24 hours. It provides a continuous recording of the ECG, during which patients record their symptoms and activities. This form of monitoring can help identify dysrhythmias as the source of the patient's lightheadedness. Antiarrhythmia drugs can then be prescribed, and the Holter monitor test repeated to monitor effectiveness of the drugs.

## Electrophysiologic study

In cases in which lightheadedness is caused by dysrhythmias, electrophysiologic testing (EPS) may be used. Patients may be mildly sedated to minimize anxiety and be given local anesthesia at the site where a catheter, with several electrodes at the distal end, is manipulated through the venous system into the right side of the heart. With electrodes in place, electrical impulses are generated in an attempt to stimulate the heart and reproduce the abnormal rhythm as recorded on the ECG. The characteristics of the dysrhythmia are analyzed for frequency, conduction path, and onset. Consequently, the appropriate pharmacologic agent can be tried. EPS may be repeated once the drug is in therapeutic range to confirm its efficacy (see Ch. 7).

# MEDICAL-SURGICAL INTERVENTION

# Pharmacology

Lightheadedness caused by ischemia-induced ectopy is managed as a symptom of CAD. Agents such as β blockers, nitrates, calcium channel blockers, and antihypertensives, which act to reduce myocardial oxygen demands, are used (see Table 4.7). When ectopy is caused by conduction tissue abnormalities, antiarrhythmic drugs are used to minimize the dysrhythmias (see Table 7.2).

Lightheadedness associated with hypotension in the absence of primary heart disease is usually managed conservatively with supine position and fluid replacement. The latter may be orally or intravenously administered. Occasionally, atropine may be used for its parasympatholytic action to raise cardiac output by increasing heart rate.

Drug-induced hypotension can cause a patient to complain of lightheadedness. The actions of antihypertensive drugs can result in an abnormally low blood pressure. For example, too great a reduction in blood volume through vigorous diuresis or excessive reduction in afterload by vasodilating agents such as prazosin or angiotensin II inhibitors may cause lightheadedness. Usually, this problem is rectified by volume replacement or by waiting for drug absorption (see Tables 4.6 and 4.7).

Lightheadedness in diabetic patients usually means they are in a hypoglycemic state. Glucose metabolism may be regulated with several pharmacological agents.

When diet therapy alone does not adequately maintain blood glucose levels in Type II diabetes mellitus, oral sulfonylureas such as orinase, diabinase, tolinase, or gliberide can be used. These generally lower hyperglycemic conditions, but may not bring blood glucose levels to normal. Sulfonylureas act by stimulating insulin production, increasing the number of insulin receptors, and improving glucose disposal. It should be noted that when these drugs are taken in combination with alcohol, the patient may complain of marked flushing around the face as well as diaphoresis.

Insulin administration can normalize blood glucose levels; however regulation of the dosage can be tedious. Regimens of drug injections are individualized according to the patient's lifestyle, food intake, weight, and ability to monitor blood or urine glucose levels. Greater insulin is required when a meal higher than usual in carbohydrates is ingested or when the patient is under greater emotional stress. Conversely, lower dosages are required for the support of both acute and habitual vigorous exercise.

## Rehabilitation

When lightheadedness is due to CAD, a graded rehabilitation program (as described in Ch. 4 and in profile 1, the case of a patient with a below knee amputation) is prescribed. In the acute recovery after a cardiac event, patients may experience lightheadedness due to prolonged bed rest. Antihypertensive drugs and the lack of gravitational stimuli can cause a decrease in vasomotor tone and lowering of peripheral vascular resistance. Active exercises performed in bed help maintain efficient circulation and minimize blood volume loss and muscle atrophy. Short periods of upright position such as dangling or sitting in a chair stimulate autonomic nervous system reflex activity to maintain blood pressure in response to gravity. External leg supports may assist in maintaining greater pressure in the lower extremities, elevating blood pressure to increase afterload. Active exercise while sitting also helps maintain blood pressure by enhancing preload. When an irregular heart beat is the cause of lightheadedness, the rhythm must be stabilized before beginning an exercise conditioning program. There is some evidence showing that aerobic exercise decreases the frequency of ventricular ectopy and may even raise the threshold for ventricular fibrillation. Relaxation techniques and counseling in stress management may also reduce dysrhythmia production (See Ch. 7).

When lightheadedness is associated with cerebrovascular insufficiency, sensorimotor deficits may be present. Rehabilitation procedures may then include neuromuscular facilitation, functional and gait training and endurance exercise. Emotional support for the patient and family and an educational program of risk factor identification and behavior modification are important components of a total rehabilitation program.

When lightheadedness is brought on by hypoglycemia and diabetes mellitis is the pathological cause, rehabilitation will depend upon the type of diabetic patient needing intervention. Diabetes mellitus is subdivided into Type I juvenile onset and Type II adult onset. Type I is always insulin dependent, can be underweight, and may be "brittle" with easily broken bones, retinopathy, neuropathy, and generalized atherosclerosis. They lack tactile perception and often have foot or hand injuries which do not heal quickly. Type II diabetics are most often obese and may not require insulin therapy, since dietary control is usually adequate for glucose metabolism if the patient is cooperative.[2] For both types, rehabilitation should include:

1. emotional support to enhance cooperation and to help deal with physical disabilities
2. education about diet, weight reduction, exercise, insulin delivery, and foot care
3. exercise to enhance glucose metabolism through physical fitness. Physically fit diabetics use insulin more efficiently and therefore require less of it.[3]

Also when ideal body weight is maintained, through diet and exercise, insulin may not be necessary even if it once was.

## Invasive Monitoring

Lightheadedness does not need invasive monitoring under usual circumstances. However, when it is caused by hypovolemia in a patient with ventricular dysfunction, fluid replacement may need to be monitored with a Swan-Ganz catheter to avoid fluid overload (See Ch. 4, Chest Pain, Invasive Monitoring).

## Invasive Procedures

Relief from lightheadedness reflects successful management of the associated diagnosis. Lightheadedness caused by ectopy indicates that treatment of the conduction abnormality will relieve the symptom. Invasive procedures such as ablation therapy, aneurysmectomy, pacemaker therapy, and use of an automatic implantable defibrillator are possible options and are described in Ch. 7.

---

## PHYSICAL THERAPY INTERVENTION

## Interview

Add these key questions to the generic interview found in Chapter 3:

1. Do you ever faint?
2. Are there any other symptoms at the same time, like nausea, chills, pain, breathlessness, blurred vision or sweating?
3. How often does this happen?
4. Are there any activities that bring it on?
5. What do you do to relieve this symptom?

## Evaluation

### Musculoskeletal Evaluation

See general physical therapy evaluation. Check neck range of motion. Check for hemiparesis with manual muscle tests.

For diabetic patients, a foot sensory evaluation should be done prior to initiating an exercise program.

### Cardiopulmonary Evaluation

See general physical therapy evaluation (see Ch. 3).

Inspection
   Look for JVD
   Look for cardiac apical pulsation
   Look for obesity vs. normal vs. under weight
   Look for trophic changes of skin, especially feet and ankles
Palpation
   Palpate for PMI
   Check peripheral pulses
   Check for skin temperatures
   Check for pitting edema

Vital Signs

**Heart Rate.** If the heart rate is inadequate to maintain an effective cardiac output, the patient can become lightheaded as when reduction in stroke volume is associated with a bradycardia, or when filling time is too short as with a sinus tachycardia.

**Heart Rhythm.** Certain dysrhythmias cause lightheadedness but only if they compromise stroke volume. The more severe the ventricular dysfunction, the less the tolerance to the dysrhythmias and the more the likelihood of lightheadedness and other symptoms (see Ch. 7).

**Blood Pressure.** Owing to gravitational effects on the circulatory system, as a patient changes position from supine to sitting to standing, a 10-mmHg drop in systolic blood pressure may be noted. This drop usually occurs without symptoms as the body quickly compensates to ensure no reduction in cardiac output. In patients on prolonged bed rest or on antihypertensive drug therapy, there may be either no reflexive increase in heart rate or a sluggish vasomotor response. These patients may incur larger drops in blood pressure and often experience lightheadedness.

Performance of a Valsalva maneuver may stimulate a drop in blood pressure and cause lightheadedness. When a subject strains against a closed airway, there is an increase in intrathoracic pressure. This limits passive filling of the heart, causing a momentary reduction in preload and therefore in blood pressure. An intact autonomic nervous system allows a reflex increase in peripheral vascular resistance as a compensatory attempt to maintain blood pressure. Once the strain is released, there is an acute increase in blood pressure due to the normal return of blood volume (preload) and the higher afterload. This is only a temporary "overshoot." If the autonomic nervous system response is insufficient, the drop in blood pressure may be sustained and there may not be any acute rise after release of the strain.

**Respiratory Rate.** Lightheadedness can be a direct result of hyperventilation due to a respiratory alkalosis. The mechanism has been explained in this chapter in connection with physical examination.

## Electrocardiogram

The ECG rhythm strip should be used to assess a possible dysrhythmia that is not being well tolerated by a patient reporting lightheadedness (see Ch. 7).

## Functional Evaluation

Orthostatic intolerance is the most common cause of lightheadedness in patients, especially in those who have been on prolonged bed rest or have had prolonged anesthesia for surgery. A functional evaluation at the point of getting a patient up out of bed for the first time consists of monitoring blood pressure and heart rate initially in supine position. When the patient is brought to sitting position, repetition of these measurements should show the adequacy of the hemodynamic adjustment. With dangling, a significant drop in blood pressure may occur with or without compensatory tachycardia. This drop may provoke lightheadedness, and standing may even produce loss of consciousness.

Another possible cause of lightheadedness is hypoxia, especially with hyperventilation. The use of finger or ear oximetry during functional activities such as walking or stair climbing or during an exercise test will help to determine whether desaturation of hemoglobin occurs with the added metabolic demand for $O_2$. The 12- or 6-minute walk test described in Chapter 5 is a more standard way to determine the significance of the lightheadedness.

Exercise programming for aerobic conditioning of the diabetic patient is done by individualized exercise prescription. An ETT should be performed to rule out CAD. If positive, the program is exactly as described for patients with CAD (see Ch. 4). If negative, an exercise intensity can be set to 70 to 85 percent of maximum functional capacity or age-predicted heart rate. Principles of aerobic conditioning should be followed: frequency: at least 3 times per week: duration: 20 to 30 minutes of high intensity exercise: mode: dynamic use of any large muscles. It may be worth noting that in these authors' experience, many obese diabetic patients do not enjoy exercise, and may need to find activities which keep them compliant.

# REFERENCES

1. Widmann F: Clinical Interpretation of Laboratory Tests. p. 45. In Endocrine Glands. F A Davis, Philadelphia, 1983
2. Ganong W: The Pancreas: Carbohydrate Metabolism. p. 269. In Review of Medical Physiology. 8th ed. Lange Medical Publishers, California, 1977
3. Costill D: Interaction of Skeletal Muscle Metabolism and Hyperlipidemia in Diabetics''. p. 97. In Pollock M and Schmidt D: (eds) Heart Disease and Rehabilitation. Houghton-Mifflin Professional Publishers, Boston, 1979

# SUGGESTED READINGS

Beebe C: Utilizing Self-monitoring of Blood Glucose in Nutrition Intervention: Catching up with Technology. Diabetes Care Educ Newsletter 8(3):1, 1987
Brown D: A Physical Therapist's Guide to Diabetes Mellitus. Cardiopulmonary Record 1(2):4, 1986
Conn, H (ed): Current Diagnosis. WB Saunders, Philadelphia, 1985
Fischer B: Techniques and Tools for Self-monitoring of Blood Glucose. Diabetes Care and Educ Newletter 8(3):2 1987
Franz M: Exercise and the Management of Diabetes mellitus, J Amer Diet Assoc 87(7):872, July 1987
Ganong W: Review of Medical Physiology, 8th ed. Lange Medical Publishers, California, 1977
Jensen M: Miles J: The Roles of Diet and Exercise in the Management of Patients with Insulin-dependent Diabetes Mellitus. Mayo Clin Proc 61:813, 1986

Petersdorf R, Adams R, Braunwald E, et al: Harrison's Principles of Internal Medicine, 10th ed. McGraw-Hill, New York, 1983

Powers, M, Interpreting and using self-blood glucose monitoring in Diabetes Care and Educ Newsletter 8(3):11, 1987

Sokolow M, McIlroy M: Clinical Cardiology. Lange Medical Publishers, California, 1981

Widmann F: Clinical Interpretation of Laboratory Tests. F A Davis, Philadelphia, 1983

Zinman B: Zuniga-Guajardo S: Kelly D: Comparison of the Acute and Long-Term Effects of Exercise and Glucose Control in Type I Diabetes. Diabetes Care, 7(6):515, Nov–Dec 1984

# LOSS OF CONSCIOUSNESS 9

Loss of consciousness may be caused by one of many mechanisms; some of these are listed in Table 9.1, which summarizes differential diagnoses. Note that the term *syncope* is synonymous with loss of consciousness. It is also important to note that there is a continuum of severity. Patients recover from vasovagal syncope spontaneously, while ventricular tachycardia and fibrillation require immediate medical intervention, including cardiopulmonary resuscitation (CPR).

## CHART REVIEW

When the patient loses consciousness during a physical therapy program, the response of the therapist must be immediate. However, it is important to note from an initial chart review any mention of a history of loss of consciousness and any description of such an event, as well as any discussion of cause. Knowledge of previous episodes will prepare the therapist for the most appropriate immediate response.

### Implications for Physical Therapy

If there is a past history of loss of consciousness, find what the precipitating cause was judged to be. Before treating the patient take the following measures in order to anticipate any loss of consciousness that may be expected.

1.  Take the blood pressure (BP). If it is low, use Ace bandages on lower extremities. Give extra water to drink. Have patient do ankle pumps before changing position.
2.  Take the heart rate. If pulse is irregular, check for previous electrocardiogram (ECG) and Holter monitoring to identify type and frequency of dysrhythmia. Compare current frequency with previous record. Use

**Table 9.1 Differential Diagnosis of Loss of Consciousness**

| Possible Causes | Possible Findings | Stimuli | Pathology |
|---|---|---|---|
| Vasovagal syncope | Hypotension, bradycardia, tinnitus, pallor, diaphoresis, rapid recovery in supine position | Fear<br>Sight of blood<br>High anxiety state | None |
| Orthostatic hypotension | Hypotension upon rising, normotension in recumbency, compensatory tachycardia | Rapid change from recumbency to upright<br>Prolonged standing<br>Hypovolemia | Loss of smooth muscle tone in veins |
| Ventricular tachycardia (VT) | Decreased blood pressure, may or may not feel pulse, ECG shows VT | Exercise<br>Electrocution<br>Spontaneous<br>Low potassium<br>Myocardial ischemia<br>Conduction disease | CAD<br>Ventricular aneurysm |
| Ventricular fibrillation (VF) | No pulse, no pressure, can see seizure, pallor, respiratory arrest, rarely conscious. ECG shows VF | Exercise<br>MI<br>VT<br>Ischemia<br>Abnormal cardiac conduction<br>Low potassium<br>Prolonged Q-T interval | CAD<br>Ventricular aneurysm |
| Asystole | No pulse, no pressure, pallor, respiratory arrest, not conscious; ECG shows flat line or unconducted P waves | MI<br>VF<br>Ischemia<br>Abnormal conduction<br>High potassium | CAD<br>CHF |

| | | | |
|---|---|---|---|
| Cardiac tamponade | Labile BP, rising with expiration, dropping with inspiration; falling BP and raised jugular venous pressure | Cardiac surgery<br>Myocardial wound<br>Pericardial effusion | Bleeding into pericardial sac |
| Pulmonary embolism | Sudden breathlessness, chest pain, cough, hemoptysis, apprehension, increased respiratory rate, increased heart rate, expiratory wheeze, fever | Prolonged bedrest<br>Recent surgery<br>Fracture of long bone<br>Atrial fibrillation<br>CHF<br>Recent MI | Obstruction of pulmonary arterial tree |
| Hypoxia | Cyanosis, increased heart rate, increased respiratory rate, pallor | Exercise<br>Cardiac arrest<br>Suffocation<br>Drowning | Respiratory or cardiac failure<br>COPD<br>Pneumonia<br>Pulmonary embolism<br>Seizure |
| Seizure | Muscle jerking; breath-holding; choking sounds, cyanotic; increased heart rate, blood pressure, respiratory rate; increased body temperature; momentary vs. minutes of loss of bladder, bowel control; tongue biting | Flickering lights<br>Loud noise<br>Chemical imbalance<br>Hypoxia<br>Time of day<br>Fatigue<br>Anxiety | Epilepsy |
| Hypoglycemia | Diaphoresis, ketone breath | Low blood sugar<br>Vigorous exercise | Diabetes mellitus |

rhythm strip to compare current dysrhythmia with previous record (see Ch. 7).

3. Check with patients having a history of seizures for auras and drug control, and make sure they have taken their usual medicine.

4. Check with diabetic patients on when they take insulin, what they experience if they need sugar or are low on insulin, and what they take for immediate sugar (see Ch. 8.)

5. If a patient has a recent history of respiratory decompensation, use oximetry during activities for measure of oxygen saturation.

## PHYSICAL THERAPY INTERVENTION

If the physical therapist is prepared for a loss of consciousness based on a history, then the physical therapy evaluation and treatment are as follows:

1. Establish unresponsiveness
   If vasovagal syncope of short duration, assist the patient to supine position
   If orthostatic intolerance of short duration, assist the patient to supine position
   If seizure, wait, monitor vital signs, and get help if prolonged
2. If unresponsive, then initiate CPR procedure
   Call for help
   Open airway if no air movement
   Deliver two quick breaths
   Check carotid pulse, if absent
   Begin cardiac compressions (15 at a time)
   Breathe two breaths between every 15 compressions
3. Certified person initiates advanced cardiac life support (ACLS) if indicated[1]
   Deliver $O_2$ with breaths, using face mask or bag-mask system
   Monitor ECG to identify rhythm:
       Ventricular fibrillation—defibrillate (see Fig. 9.1)
       Ventricular tachycardia—defibrillate or suppress with lidocaine (see Fig. 9.2)
       Asystole—epinephrine and lidocaine
       Bradycardia—atropine and isoproterenol
   Intravenous access for drug administration
   Intubate for ventilation and/or drug administration
4. Continue CPR until arrhythmia abates, consciousness returns, and patient recovers

*Note*: It is important to become certified in CPR and ACLS by the

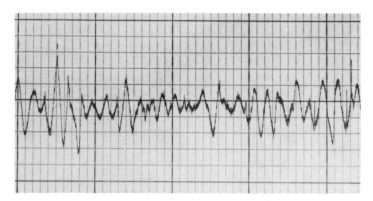

**Fig. 9.1** Ventricular fibrillation. (Reproduced from Thys D, Kaplan J: The ECG in Anesthesia and Critical Care. p. 164. Churchill Livingstone, New York, 1987, with permission).

American Heart Association certification or American Red Cross, in order to properly perform these procedures.

## Patient Examples

Examples of patients who may lose consciousness and require a full "code" procedure include those who have ventricular ectopy, which indicates highly irritable ventricles and susceptibility to the following dangerous dysrhythmias:

Premature ventricular contractions (PVCs) more often than 6 per minute which increase in frequency during activity

PVCs from several foci (multiform)

PVCs occurring on the T wave of a previous QRS-T complex (R on T phenomenon), causing ventricular tachycardia (see Ch. 7).

Patients who have had an anterior myocardial infarction (MI) are at

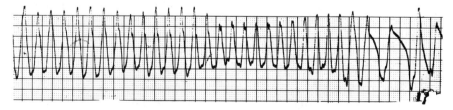

**Fig. 9.2** Ventricular tachycardia. (Reproduced from Thys D, Kaplan J: The ECG in Anesthesia and Critical Care. p. 163. Churchill Livingstone, New York, 1987, with permission).

higher risk for ventricular aneurysm and therefore for a greater degree of ventricular dysfunction. This may result in a very low ejection fraction, which permits very little cardiac reserve. Myocardial ischemia will most likely occur at very low levels of work.

Patients who have had a posterior MI are at higher risk for papillary muscle dysfunction. Disruption of the papillary muscle chordae tendineae will produce mitral insufficiency. Mitral regurgitation may produce pulmonary edema, which may be sudden and fulminating when the mitral valve tendon is torn.

Patients who have chronic obstructive pulmonary disease (COPD) with a large component of chronic bronchitis (the "blue bloater" appearance) also often have a large degree of right ventricular strain due to long-standing pulmonary hypertension with hypoxia and hypercapnia. Their partial pressure of oxygen in arterial blood ($PaO_2$) is lower than normal (95 mmHg) and may be as low as 60 or below, an indication for supplemental $O_2$. Their partial pressure of carbon dioxide in arterial blood ($PaCO_2$) is higher than normal (40 mmHg), indicating $CO_2$ retention. This in turn blunts the normal drive to breathe despite the metabolic buffer of the pH. These patients may have chronic cor pulmonale for years and may exhibit irregular heart beats, especially atrial arrhythmias such as occasional premature atrial contractions, atrial flutter, or atrial fibrillation; PVCs are also frequent and may lead to serious complications. The loss of consciousness problem would most likely be due to left-sided heart failure, occurring as a consequence of right-sided failure with severe wheezing, breathlessness, and the possibility of respiratory arrest and ventricular fibrillation.

Patients who are neurologically unstable owing to recent cerebrovascular accident, head trauma, or other central nervous system insult, often exhibit new dysrhythmias during the period of instability. These may be due to elevation of intracranial pressure, and once this has been controlled and returned to normal range, dysrhythmias usually disappear. However, in patients who have pre-existing dysrhythmias, pre-existing coronary artery disease (CAD), or congestive heart failure (CHF), these "transient dysrhythmias" may not disappear and may lead to serious complications. Dizziness and loss of consciousness may occur, due not to "transient ischemic attacks," which are often suspected, but to loss of brain perfusion when the dysrhythmia results in a serious reduction in cardiac output. Transient dysrhythmias are usually not treated with antiarrhythmic medications. The physical therapist working with stroke patients in the early recovery period should monitor patients by pulse-taking for these dysrhythmias, and if they are palpated, should apply a simple ECG single-lead monitor to identify the dysrhythmia. New dysrhythmias should be reported to the physician, with documentation by ECG strip. The physical therapist may be the first health care worker to identify a dysrhythmia in some patients, especially those whose dysrhythmia appears during exercise.

# REFERENCE

1. Montgomery WH, Donegan J, McIntyre K: Standards and guidelines for cardio-pulmonary resuscitation and emergency cardiac care. JAMA 255: 2915, 1986

# SUGGESTED READING

McIntyre K, Lewis J (eds): Textbook of Advanced Cardiac Life Support. American Heart Association, Dallas, 1983

# COUGH 10

Cough is a protective reflexive maneuver and thus valuable to the organism. It occurs in order to expel from the large airways material that potentially could obstruct air flow and cause asphyxiation or choking; yet it can become chronic, ineffective, and annoying. Rarely should a cough be suppressed. Treatment for cough is most often geared toward enhancing cough effectiveness; thus assistance with clearing airways makes it easier for patients to use cough effectively. There are multiple causes of cough, as outlined in Table 10.1, and treatment must be aimed at specific causes.

## CHART REVIEW

In the chart review the physical examination, history, vital signs, pertinent test results, and interventions should be analyzed.

## Medical History

The history should be used to ascertain the cough frequency, the sound of the cough, how long the current cough symptom has endured, what triggers the cough, and when or during which activities, such as eating, the cough occurs or is worse. Are there accompanying sounds or complaints with the cough, such as hoarseness, stridor, or wheeze? Is the cough productive of sputum? If so, what is the description of the sputum? Consider its quantity, color, odor, and consistency. The patient's smoking history is relevant here, and in the case of a current smoker, the cough is certainly related to the constant irritation to the airway. The patient may have been exposed to environmental airway irritants, air pollutants, asbestos, dust, etc. There may be a relevant family history for lung cancer or emphysema.

### Implication for Physical Therapy

If cough has appeared frequently in the past, this suggests the need for a complete pulmonary evaluation and possible pulmonary hygiene. See Physical Therapy Intervention below and Chapter 5.

**Table 10.1 Differential Diagnosis of Cough**

| Possible causes | Possible Finding | Stimulus | Pathology |
| --- | --- | --- | --- |
| Left ventricular dysfunction (including mitral valve dysfunction) | Bibasilar rales; breathlessness; cardiomegaly; Kerley B lines<br>Cough: bubbling, loose, rattling<br>Sputum: frothy, pink | Exercise<br>Metabolic stress<br>Supine position<br>Paroxysmal nocturnal dyspnea (PND) | Pulmonary edema<br>Left ventricular CHF |
| Bronchospasm | Wheezes, inspiratory and expiratory; increased A-P chest diameter<br>Cough: hacking, tight, spasmodic<br>Sputum: mucus plugs, mucoid tan | Exercise<br>Airborne allergens<br>Cold air<br>Anxiety<br>Upper respiratory tract infection | Asthma |
| Infection of lung | Fever; decreased breath sounds; diaphoresis; increased density on chest x-ray<br>Cough: painful, dry or productive; paroxysmal<br>Sputum: dark, green, thick, can be odorous, rusty color, mucoid or blood-tinged | Microbes<br>Immunosuppression<br>Atelectasis | Pneumonia |
| Inflammation of lung | Rhonchi; breathlessness; wheezing; pain; fatigue<br>Cough: variable, persistent<br>Sputum: purulent, copious | Airborne irritants<br>Upper respiratory tract infection<br>Asthma<br>Allergy<br>Smoke inhalation<br>Lung infarction<br>Aspiration | Sarcoidosis<br>Infection<br>Allergic reaction<br>Pneumonitis |
| | Sputum: can be layered, hemoptysis can occur, can be foul-smelling | Chronic airway infections<br>Radiation | Bronchiectasis |

| Pathophysiology | Signs/Symptoms | Cause | Condition |
|---|---|---|---|
| Overproduction of mucous glands | Barrel chest; finger clubbing; hypoxia and cyanosis<br>*Cough:* frequent, productive, labored<br>*Sputum:* purulent, green, mucoid, copious | Genetic | Cystic fibrosis |
| Obstruction to air flow, gas exchange | Decreased breath sounds; breathlessness; weight loss; appetite loss; chest x-ray shows lesion; fatigue<br>*Cough:* shallow, persistent, sometimes painful<br>*Sputum:* can be of any description | Genetic (?) cell mutation | Lung tumor |
| | Breath sounds with any adventitious sounds; breathlessness; fatigue; use of accessory muscles; bullae on chest x-ray; increased A-P chest diameter<br>*Cough:* A.M., can be loose, or tight<br>*Sputum:* sparse or copious, mucoid, white to yellow | Chronic smoking<br>Genetic (?)<br>Repeated upper respiratory tract infections | Chronic obstructive pulmonary disease, especially chronic bronchitis |
| Choking | No vocalization; panic; cyanosis; wheezing; rib retraction; nasal flaring<br>*Cough:* marked effort, stridor<br>*Sputum:* none | Foreign body or tongue in airway | None |
| Alveolar collapse | Decreased $PO_2$, decreased breath sounds<br>*Cough:* honking<br>*Sputum:* none or consistent with a coexistent pathology | Hypoventilation<br>After surgery/anesthesia<br>Decreased mobility<br>Restrictive lung disease<br>Neuromuscular dysfunction | Atelectasis |
| Aging of scarred lung tissue | *Cough:* persistent, nonproductive<br>*Sputum:* none | Radiation therapy<br>History of pneumonia | Interstitial fibrosis |

## Physical Examination

### Vital Signs

Cough alone should not disturb vital signs except when associated with a fever. However, respiratory rhythm may be disturbed by cough, and breath sounds may include wheeze, rhonchi, and rales.

## Tests

### Laboratory Values

Arterial Blood Gases

See Chapter 5.

Complete Blood Count

A complete blood count will help determine the presence of respiratory infection, as indicated by an elevated white cell count (see Ch. 6).

Chest x-Ray

X-ray findings will show infection ("white out") and will show an enlarged silhouette of the heart in congestive heart failure (CHF) ("the boot shape"). They will show the chronic hyperinflation changes of the patient with emphysema and/or chronic bronchitis, including barrel chest and low, flattened diaphragm. They will show foreign bodies in airways in some cases and may assist in showing tumor. Angiography of the pulmonary vasculature will show pulmonary embolus (see Ch. 5).

Pulmonary Function Tests

Evaluation of chronic cough will include pulmonary function tests to determine the presence and extent of airway obstruction. Flow characteristics may be diminished, as shown by reduction of 1-second forced expiratory volume ($FEV_1$) (see Ch. 5).

Sputum Culture

A sputum analysis is done to determine what organisms can be grown in a culture medium from the sputum. This helps to determine whether bacterial infection is present and if so which antibiotic may be best for attacking specific bacteria. Viral infections are not treated with antibiotics.

Common organisms causing primary lung infection include:

Pneumococci
Staphylococci
Streptococci

*Klebsiella* spp.
Gram-negative intestinal bacilli
*Haemophilus influenzae*
*Francisella tularensis*
*Mycoplasma*
Rickettsiae
*Chlamydia psittaci*
Fungi
*Pneumocystis carinii*

## Cough Effectiveness

A single measurement of expiratory peak flow can easily be made with a Wright peak flow meter or an electronic spirometer. Since cough effectiveness is primarily determined by the patient's ability to generate a high, abrupt, forceful expiratory flow in order to expectorate, this measurement is singularly valuable for the determination of cough effort efficacy. It is not often made on a routine basis but it is simple to perform. Information obtained from this measurement would be especially helpful to the physical therapist facilitating cough.[1]

## Bronchoscopy

See Chapter 5.

## Laryngoscopy

A laryngoscope is a long, curved device with a flashlight on the end, which may be introduced into a patient's throat to probe to the level of the larynx in order to find foreign bodies or malformations. These devices may produce choking and coughing but can yield important information about structure, which helps to define appropriate intervention.

# MEDICAL-SURGICAL INTERVENTION

## Pharmacology

The pharmacologic interventions used for cough include antibiotics to treat underlying disease that produces unusual cough symptoms in conjunction with x-ray findings, sputum changes, and often fever. These antibiotics are listed in Table 5.7. For cough treatment three specific types of agents may be employed: expectorants, mucolytic agents, and antitussives (Table 10.2). The last are used only in very circumspect cases when a cough is chronic and nonproductive and is itself more of an irritant than it is a help.

Table 10.2 Drugs Used in the Treatment of Cough

| Drug Category | Actions |
|---|---|
| Expectorants: | |
| Guaifenesin | Decreases viscosity of tenacious secretions |
| Hydriodic acid | Liquefies thick, tenacious sputum |
| | Used in chronic bronchitis, asthma |
| Iodinated glycerol | Liquefies thick, tenacious secretions |
| Potassium iodide | Increases respiratory tract secretions |
| | Decreases viscosity |
| Mucolytic agents | |
| Acetylcysteine | Decreases viscosity of pulmonary secretions |
| | Decreases disulfide linkages of mucoproteins |
| Antitussives | |
| Benzonatate | Inhibits cough production by anesthetizing cough–sensitive sites (vagal afferent fibers in bronchi, alveoli, pleurae) |
| Codeine | Symptomatic relief of nonproductive cough |
| Dextromethorphan | In chronic, nonproductive cough accompanied by minor throat and bronchial irritation provides relief like codeine |

## Humidity and Warmth

It is important for the purpose of successful expectoration to keep sputum moist. Patients need to be encouraged to drink water (8 to 12 glasses per day) and, if tolerated, to use humidifiers in dry air environments. Without this precaution sputum becomes very sticky and difficult to move.

# Rehabilitation

Principles of rehabilitation are the same as those outlined for breathlessness in Chapter 5.

# Invasive Monitoring

Although invasive monitoring may be necessary for many conditions in which cough is a symptom, there are no specific monitoring needs for cough per se.

# Invasive Procedures

## Suctioning

Suctioning is the introduction of a small-gauge suction catheter into the airway under sterile conditions with the purpose of removing tenacious secretions. Suctioning is only done when a cough is ineffective and is considered to be the major cough-enhancing and secretion removal technique available. Suctioning should be a sterile technique. The size of the suction catheter depends upon the size of the patient; normal adults require most commonly a #14 French catheter. Suctioning may be by nasopharyngeal, oropharyngeal, or endotracheal tube or via a tracheostomy. The technique requires a period of preoxygenation with 100 percent oxygen, should never be used for longer than 10 to 15 seconds at a time, and should be applied intermittently. It should always be followed by a maximal sustained breath-holding maneuver or, by use of an ambu bag, by maximal ventilation to provide for adequate reventilation of all areas of the lung. Suctioning is usually performed with the head of the bed elevated by 45°. The hazards of suctioning include: the introduction of infectious organisms into sterile lung fields; the drop in blood oxygenation inherent in the period of nonbreathing while suctioning is carried out; the possibility of low perfusion states, which may precipitate cardiac arrhythmias and loss of consciousness; and the possibility of suctioning out lung parenchyma rather than only airway contents.

Another invasive procedure that does stimulate a cough but is not performed for the express purpose of cough stimulation is bronchoscopy, discussed in Chapter 5.

## PHYSICAL THERAPY INTERVENTION

## Interview

Add these key questions to the generic physical therapy patient interview found in Chapter 3:

1. Do you get short of breath when you cough?
2. Is your cough productive in bringing up phlegm?
3. What are the color, consistency, and quantity of your phlegm?
4. Is there some usual time of day when you cough?
5. Do you ever stifle your cough? If so, why?

## Evaluation

In addition to the generic physical therapy evaluation, a cough evaluation and chest evaluation may be made. If the primary cause of the cough can be ascertained (lung disease) and if postural drainage, manual techniques, and cough enhancement are indicated by examination of breath sounds and cough effectiveness, then treatment geared toward airway clearance may be extremely effective.

### Cough Evaluation

Force of Cough

Make sure that the patient gets a full breath behind each cough effort and that each effort involves one or two deep, strong coughs. No long sustained coughs that become shallow should be permitted. The wheezing, tight cough of airway collapse should also be discouraged. Sometimes preceding each cough effort by short strong huffs, two at a time, helps the cough to be more effective.

Productivity of Cough

The amount of sputum and its color, consistency, and odor, if present, should be noted.

## Functional Evaluation

The 6-minute walk test with ear or finger oximetry to determine oxygen saturation is an effective objective measure of a patient's functional capacity (see Ch. 5). During coughing the patient should try not to stop the walk but to achieve a rapidly effective cough and continue walking. When a cough is "spastic," sustained, and fatiguing, it can limit the walk to shorter distances. It can also result in airway collapse causing difficulty in breathing air in as well as out. A drop in oxygen saturation may occur with this type of cough. For these reasons cough retraining is a very important physical therapy intervention.

Cough Rehabilitation

Since the cough reflex requires an intact sensitivity to tracheal stimulation as well as a powerful muscular response mechanism capable of generating very high intrathoracic pressures to forcefully expel sputum, a test of the reflex by tracheal "tickle" may be needed. Either a tonsil-tip catheter to stimulate the back of the throat with light tickle or a short but powerful pressure applied over the cricoid membrane to tickle the trachea may produce a cough. A cough response should recruit a deep inspiration and produce a forceful, visible contraction of abdominal wall muscles. A patient with weak or nonfunctional abdominal muscles (e.g., quadriplegics and abdominal surgery postoperative patients with pain) may need splinting or powerful abdominal thrusts by a helper to achieve an adequate cough. Many patients benefit by a vigorous program of abdominal wall strengthening exercise to help a weak cough become strong and effective.

## REFERENCE

1. Sciaky A: Predictors of Postoperative Ability to Clear Pulmonary Secretion. Unpublished Master's Thesis, MGH Institute of Health Professions at the MA. General Hospital, 1987

# LEG PAIN

# 11

Patient descriptors and history are key to the differential diagnosis of the complaint of leg pain. Peripheral vascular disease (PVD), either of arterial or venous origin, frequently occurs concurrently with coronary artery disease (CAD) and is often found in elderly patients. The pain of PVD can be more debilitating than angina or breathlessness in some patients, and for the unfortunate ones who experience all of these symptoms rehabilitation is imperative (Table 11.1).

## CHART REVIEW

Chart review is important for this symptom. Location of leg pain may be very specific, may be generalized, or may have changed over a period of time.

## Medical History

In the written history look for duration of symptoms, date of onset of intermittent claudication or other leg pain, triggers for the pain (i.e., what specific activities bring it on—shin splints are highly specific, whereas muscle ischemia relates to length or level of exertion), and what brings relief (position, rest). Note associated diagnoses such as CAD or diabetes mellitus. Check for vocational or avocational history. For example, an occupation requiring long hours of standing over years may produce venous stasis problems, while an athlete may have shin splints, or anterior compartment syndrome (see case profile 5, which describes an athlete with exercise-induced asthma). Is there any smoking history? Evidence for hyperlipidemia? Not many charts will report skin temperature maps, but there are facilities where thermography is done to map the arterial distribution of a limb. Always note the presence or absence of peripheral pulses or the strength of the palpable pulses. Specific word descriptors of pain can be most helpful to differentiate among the many possible diagnoses causing the pain. The presence of pitting edema along with pain is usually associated with vascular disease.[1]

**Table 11.1 Differential Diagnosis of Leg Pain**

| Possible Causes | Possible Findings | Stimulus | Pathology |
|---|---|---|---|
| Muscle ischemia Anterior compartment syndrome | Pain (cramp) increases with exertion; local pain grows sharper; stops with rest; weakness | Walking; running | Connective tissue tightness |
| Intermittent claudication Shin splints | Anterior pain on any dorsiflexion; local tenderness to pressure; ache; soreness; x-ray may show bone abnormality | Overuse; jogging; running; walking | Peripheral vascular disease Microtearing of muscle fibers; stress fractures; periosteal separation; periostitis |
| Joint pain Arthritis, degenerative joint disease | Pain on motion of joint or weight-bearing; pain may be acute, sharp; x-ray may show arthritic joint changes | Trauma; pivoting; weight shifting; running | Inflammation, biomechanical malalignment |
| Gout | Knee, big toe; localized pain; red, hot, throbbing, searing pain; nocturnal onset; hyperuricemia | Fatigue Diuretic usage Minor trauma | Uric acid crystal accumulation in joint |
| Low back pain and sciatica | Radiating pain down back of leg; numbness; tingling; weakness; pseudoclaudication; CT scan, x-ray, myelogram show spinal column pathology | Foward flexion Prolonged sitting Bending with rotation Poor body mechanics | Spinal column pathology; herniated disc; spinal tumor; spondylolithiasis |
| Gangrene of foot | Severe, intractable, constant pain in local area; trophic changes; cold skin; blue-purple skin areas | Hypoxemia Cellular metabolites stimulating free nerve endings | Arterial obstruction |
| Venous stasis ulcer | Raw, throbbing, nauseating pain; brown-purple swollen skin; edema of ankles | Years of standing on feet | Edema Increase in venous pressure |
| Peripheral neuropathy (e.g., diabetes mellitus) | Burning, lancinating pain; trophic changes; loss of sensation in feet; reduced nerve conduction velocity | Motion Touch Cold Heat | Trauma Chronic hyperglycemia Alcoholism Inflammation |

## *Implications for Physical Therapy*

If there is any clue about the etiology from the medical history, check for related test results in the chart before treating the patient with leg pain.

# Physical Examination

## *Physical Appearance*

The patient with leg pain may have no change in physical appearance. However, when there is a vascular etiology, there may be skin discoloration and trophic changes. For example, venous stasis produces brown, swollen areas on foot or ankle, and arterial insufficiency produces shiny, atrophic skin with no hair growth. Eventually, skin may turn blue or purple with chronic arterial obstruction.[1]

## *Vital Signs*

Note core temperature, peripheral pulses, and any record of skin temperatures. If skin is cool, suspect vascular obstruction. If hot, suspect active inflammation or infection.

# Tests

## *Laboratory Values*

### Uric Acid

Blood tests may include uric acid level to assess the presence and severity of gout, which is marked by a higher than expected level of uric acid. Crystals precipitate into specific joints, resulting in the typical pattern of gout-type pain in the big toe or the knee joint (see Appendix for normal values).

### Glucose Testing

See Chapter 8.

## *Tests for Circulatory Insufficiency*

### Doppler Velocity Detection

Doppler flowmeters are used in a noninvasive test to determine blood flow through an artery. They are used along the anatomic course of a specific artery and are useful in the larger, superficial arteries of the body, such as the carotid or the femoral. A continuous ultrasonic beam is passed through an artery and across the column of blood. It is picked up on a receiving transducer. The rate and direction of blood flow causes frequency shifts in the sound beam. Frequency changes can be used to estimate arterial obstruction.

One application of a Doppler velocity detector is in the measurement of segmental extremity pressure. A sphygmomanometer cuff is applied to the thigh and/or the calf. The Doppler probe is placed along the vessel being studied (e.g., the popliteal artery) as the sound detector rather than a stethoscope. The cuff is inflated to a high pressure and then slowly released, and flow is first detected at the point of systolic pressure. A gradient in pressure between two measurement sites helps to localize the segment in which arterial obstruction is significant.[2]

## Plethysmography

A pulse volume recorder (PVR) is a system used to measure the total limb volume change between systole and diastole. Three sphygmomanometers are applied at the thigh, calf, and ankle. Each is inflated to 65 mmHg, and the shift in the pressure within each cuff that occurs with systole records the pulse pressure wave. This wave is then computed into a volume measurement.

## Exercise Tests for Peripheral Vascular Disease

An exercise test is used to detect early lesions of PVD and evaluate the benefits of specific therapies, including surgery, because it permits functional measurement of the hemodynamic significance of vascular stenoses. It is useful for patients with intermittent claudication who have no report of pain at rest.

Baseline arm and ankle pressures are taken with a Doppler sensor. The PVR measures volume at the end of exercise and for a 10-minute recovery period. The patient walks on a treadmill for no more than 5 minutes at 2 mph and a 10 to 12 percent grade. This provides a low level of stress and usually is sufficient to show abnormal blood flow in the legs without producing angina or breathlessness.[3]

**Implications for Physical Therapy**

Baseline function for exercise intervention is given by exercise test. Repeat test shows improved function from exercise intervention.

Exercise limitations are defined and permit an individualized exercise prescription to be made.

## Thermography

Color charts of the temperature of a limb are generated by the technique of thermography. A temperature-sensitive chemical is painted on the skin surface and turns color according to the temperature of the skin. Painful sites may correlate most with hot spots or cold spots, depending on the etiology of the pain. A cold spot occurs where there is an insufficient arterial supply, and a hot spot occurs at a site of inflammation.[4]

Table 11.2 Diagnostic Tests For Peripheral Vascular Disease

| Purpose | Technique |
|---|---|
| Recognition of stenosis | Doppler velocity detector |
| | Plethysmography |
| Location of stenosis | Venography |
| | Angiography |
| Assessment of severity | Pulse volume recorder at rest and with exercise |
| | Reactive hyperemia |
| | Effect of heat and cold |
| | Temperature mapping |
| | Thermography, thermistors |
| | Angiography |

**Implication for Physical Therapy.** Thermography is only useful to show relative change in circulation of a body part. It will not allow a comparison of one patient with another or with a norm, but it can help measure the effectiveness of a treatment.

## Arteriogram

Peripheral arteriograms that trace a radiopaque dye as it flows through an artery or arterial tree can be very helpful in determining actual arteriosclerotic lesions in the periphery. When these plaques are discrete enough and severe, bypass surgery may be indicated. This test is done in some cases to assess the need for bypass surgery or angioplasty.[5]

## Venogram

Radiopaque dye injection into large veins can be visualized by x-ray in order to study the course of a vein. Varicosities create irregularities, or "kinks" in alignment; points of narrowing, which may be due to venospasm or to occlusion, may all be pinpointed.[6]

A summary of tests used for evaluation of PVD is shown in Table 11.2.

**Implications for Physical Therapy.** The exercise study as an assessment of severity provides functional information as well. Selection of speed and angle of incline gives intensity, and the duration of test gives a sense of "endurance" before pain stops the patient. These limits can be used to set a training intensity at the maximal level tolerated.

In the absence of special tests or exercise study the physical therapist can do a fairly reasonable assessment in the department based on reactive hyperemia produced with a blood pressure cuff. The limb is elevated and the artery is occluded by cuff inflation; following this, the cuff is released and the limb dropped to time the flush of blood returning to capillary beds of the skin. Temperature and color reactions to heat and cold are also useful to evaluate the reactiveness of the vascular beds.[1]

## MEDICAL–SURGICAL INTERVENTION

### Pharmacology

Analgesics are often useful for such conditions as shin splints of musculotendinous origin and for conditions that are not considered to be inflammatory but cause unbearable pain, such as peripheral neuropathy and in gangrene with ulceration. For gout there is a special pharmacologic intervention: allupurinol is used to prevent pain by controlling uric acid level. For muscle spasm or tension, mephrobamate or Valium or a host of other muscle relaxants may be used. Since some conditions resulting in leg pain are derived from inflammation, as with periostitis, or from overuse syndromes, nonsteroidal anti-inflammatory drugs such as ibuprofen may be used. For intermittent claudication or muscle ischemia pain, several approaches have been taken, none of which is absolutely effective. Muscle ischemia is relieved, in theory, by promoting or enhancing blood flow into capillary beds in muscles where such flow is compromised by disease such as arteriosclerosis. In some cases tissue oxygenation is enhanced by increasing the ease with which blood elements cross the critical nutrient membranes for gas exchange. This is done in a hyperbaric oxygen chamber in which $O_2$ is driven directly into local tissue.

### Invasive Monitoring

Monitoring of blood flow in legs is most often done noninvasively by use of devices such as the Doppler velocity detector, plethysmograph, PVR, and thermistor (see discussion of tests, above).

### Invasive Treatment Procedures

The most common sites of lesion-producing intermittent claudication are the iliac and distal femoral arteries. Revascularization procedures for significant stenoses include bypass surgery, either saphenous vein or synthetic graft, and transluminal angioplasty. Most frequently bypassed vessels are portions of the abdominal aorta, the femoral artery, and the celiac artery. Types of bypass surgeries performed include aortofemoral, femorofemoral, and axillofemoral bypass. More distally, the femoropopliteal and femorotibial bypasses are common. Synthetic material is sometimes used for these bypasses, but these most often are subject to early failure. Vein grafts are more successful, especially when followed up with the powerful anticlotting agent urokinase.

Angioplasty may be done when lesions are discrete, less than 5–10 cm, and in larger arteries or vein grafts. A balloon-tipped catheter is introduced into the lumen of the artery. The balloon is inflated, crushing the lesion to open the lumen size.[7]

When grafts fail and repeat grafts become impossible, amputation may be necessary owing to arterial disease.[8]

# Rehabilitation

A comprehensive treatment program for patients with PVD either pre- or postoperatively should include emotional support, education, and exercise.

## Emotional Support

Patients with PVD need support for a variety of reasons. They are experiencing a decline in their functional ability as intermittent claudication begins to limit their tolerance for walking. They are in pain when they walk. They are told that the problem they have can only get worse or stay the same, and that they may possibly need surgery in the future. Some face the prospect of amputation.

## Education

Dietary management to reduce hyperlipidemia and to help in weight reduction should be initiated. Smoking cessation is a very important intervention for this disease. Hygiene and foot care should be carefully taught to prevent gangrene. Minor trauma, poorly fitting shoes, and poor toenail clipping can easily lead to gangrene.

## Exercise

A walking program is possible in some patients, in spite of intermittent claudication, by asking them to walk distances to the point of pain intolerance at frequent intervals.[9,10] However, a stationary bicycle program is usually more tolerable for longer durations. Exercise of a low-intensity, dynamic nature helps to develop a higher mechanical efficiency for performance of the specific activity, a higher anaerobic capacity (tolerance to ischemic pain and blood lactate), and an improvement of leg muscle oxygenation. The latter may be accomplished through several mechanisms:

Improved muscle blood flow (collateralization?)
Higher arteriovenous oxygen difference locally
More local muscle capillary beds
Higher levels of oxidative enzymes[11-13]

## PHYSICAL THERAPY INTERVENTION

## Interview

Add these key questions to the generic physical therapy patient interview in Chapter 3:

1. What brings on your leg pain?
2. What do you do to relieve it?
3. Describe in your own words your pain.
4. What do you think is causing the leg pain?
5. Did you ever injure the sore leg?

## Evaluation

Add the following to generic physical therapy evaluation in Chapter 3.

### Musculoskeletal Evaluation

Leg range of motion at each joint
Manual muscle testing of leg muscles
Leg muscular endurance
Sensation: cutaneous tactile sensation, especially of ankles and feet
Skin characteristics: temperature at many sites, turgor, dryness, generalized pitting edema, open lesions, scars, color, tenderness
Leg length discrepancy

### Cardiopulmonary Evaluation

Inspection

Check for spinal deformity
Check for trophic changes of skin (including discoloration)
Check for presence of skin ulceration, gangrene

Palpation

Check for presence or absence of peripheral pulses: femoral, popliteal, tibial
Check for skin temperature and dampness or dryness
Check for pitting edema

### Functional Evaluation

Intermittent claudication is a symptom related specifically to walking. A functional walking distance can be determined so that time and distance from start to pain onset and to pain intolerance are end points. After rehabilitation or surgery this provides a repeatable measure to show progress or improvement. The speed of walking needs to be controlled for a comparison measurement.

If patients have chest pain, a diagnosis of CAD, or both, an electrocardiographic monitor should be added to the walking distance test, and blood pressure may also be measured before and after any exercise. This will help to determine whether cardiac signs or symptoms limit the functional capacity of a patient before leg pain.

## Physical Therapy Rehabilitation Program

An exercise rehabilitation program for intermittent claudication should involve low-intensity, high-repetition dynamic use of leg muscles at least once daily for a minimum of 1 hour. If this is limited by pain, the patient should go to the point of pain intolerance (e.g., walking), then resume once pain is relieved. (Using pain intolerance as the end point is a very important stimulus for improvement. It is hypothesized that hypoxia at tissue level promotes collateralization.) Even if there is no pain, the exercise should be performed for 1 hour.

If there is an ulceration or gangrene, exercise should still be performed with protective dressings. Wrapping an edematous leg with an Ace bandage assists venous return. Special physical modalities to promote healing may be useful as an adjunct to the exercise program.[14]

# REFERENCES

1. Abramson D: Circulatory Diseases of the limbs: A Primer. Grune & Stratton, Orlando, FL, 1978
2. Baker JD: The vascular laboratory. p. 139. In Moore W (ed): Vascular Surgery. A Comprehensive Review. Grune & Stratton, Orlando, FL, 1983
3. Strandness D: Exercise testing in the evaluation of patients undergoing direct arterial surgery. J Cardiovasc Surg 11:192, 1970
4. Burton A: The range and variability of the blood flow in the human fingers and the vasomotor regulation of body temperature. Am J Physiol 127:437, 1939
5. Rutherford R: Vascular Surgery. 2nd Ed. WB Saunders, Philadelphia, 1984
6. Bernstein E, Fronek A: Current status of non-invasive tests in the diagnosis of peripheral arterial disease. Surg Clin North Am 62(3): 473, 1982
7. Gomes A: Principles of Angiography, p. 217. In Moore W (ed): Vascular Surgery. A Comprehensive Review. Grune & Stratton, Orlando, FL, 1983
8. Sumner D, Strandness D: Hemodynamic studies before and after extended bypass grafts to the tibial and peroneal arteries. Surgery 86:442, 1979
9. Cash JE: Chest, Heart and Vascular Disorders for Physiotherapists. Faber & Faber, London, 1975
10. Dahllof A, Holm J, Scherstein T: Exercise training of patients with intermittent claudication. Scand J Rehabil Med [suppl.] 9:20, 1983

11. Cohen L, Mock M, Rinqvist I: Physical Training in Patients with Intermittent Claudication In Saltin B (ed): Physical Conditioning and Cardiovascular Rehabilitation. Wiley Medical Publications, New York, 1981
12. Jonason T, Jonzon B, Rinqvist I: Effect of physical training on different categories of patients with intermittent claudication. Acta Med Scand 206:253, 1979
13. Schoop W: Mechanism of beneficial action of daily walking training of patients with intermittent claudication. Scand J Clin Lab Invest [Suppl] 128:197, 1973
14. Corman L: Laboratory Investigation of peripheral artery disease. p. 491. In Atherosclerotic Vascular Disease. a Hahnemann Symposium: Appleton & Lange, East Norwalk, CT, 1967

## SUGGESTED READING

Lee K (ed): Atherosclerosis. New York Academy of Sciences, New York, 1985

# EDEMA 12

A rather simplified distinction is made between two major causes of edema in Table 12.1. To clarify these two, some further definition is needed. The reader should note that there are more than two causes in fact, but additional ones will not be presented here.

*Internal filtration pressure* refers to the pressure within a blood vessel that tends to drive gases, particles, or blood elements outward unless opposed by higher tissue pressures outside the vessel wall. Factors that elevate arterial blood pressure, including hydrostatic pressure, will determine the internal filtration pressure. Only when the hydrostatic pressure of the interstitial fluid is higher than the internal filtration pressure, which occurs in peripheral edema, will fluid flow inward into the vessel.

*Oncotic pressure* refers to an osmotic pressure gradient that is set up across the capillary membrane. Colloid osmotic pressure is determined by the amount of protein colloidal substances on either side of a membrane that exerts an attraction for water. The net pull of oncotic forces determines in which direction water will flow. Protein substances leak from their compartments when there is tissue damage and are found in some quantity, under normal conditions, in lymph channels. This drawing of water causes an increased fluid volume in the region of excess protein accumulation.

## CHART REVIEW

Swelling is such a nonspecific complaint that a careful differential assessment is critical, especially in order to ascertain whether there is a cardiovascular origin to the difficulty. Since it is a hallmark sign, accompanying additional findings, for right ventricular failure, it is a highly important finding to be aware of.

### Medical History

Determine the location of the edema. Is it in only one joint? Is it in dependent parts? Is it in a site that has a surgical scar?

What is the duration of the edema? Does it recur? Is it always in the

**Table 12.1 Differential Diagnosis of Edema**

| Possible Causes | Possible Findings | Stimulus | Pathology |
|---|---|---|---|
| Increased capillary filtration pressure (over 18 mmHg) | Vasodilation of arterioles; venular constriction; increased sodium in blood; increased blood pressure; pedal edema; distended neck veins; ascites; weight gain; "blue bloater"; anasarca | Fluid overload (local or systemic) Increased venous pressure | Cardiac surgery<br>Kidney dysfunction<br>CHF of right ventricle<br>Venous valve incompetence<br>Venous obstruction<br>Cardiac valve stenosis<br>Pulmonary hypertension<br>Cirrhosis |
| Prolonged elevated venous pressure in lower extremities | Frequent, indolent ulceration with pain; purple discoloration of skin; pedal edema, bilateral and pitting | Years of standing on feet (opposing gravity) | Venous stasis with venous valve incompetence |
| Decreased oncotic pressure | Increased urinary albumin; increased local temperature; facial puffiness | Decreased plasma protein (globulin, albumin)<br>Accumulation of colloidal substances (active metabolites)<br>Drugs (steroids, nifedipine) | Cirrhosis<br>Allergic reaction<br>Nephrosis<br>Inflammation<br>Infection<br>Burns<br>Trauma |
| Lymph incompetence | Massive edema confined to one location; can be painless; loss of ROM; can be postoperative (e.g., mastectomy) | Surgery<br>Neoplasm | Obstruction of lymph channel |
| Left ventricular CHF producing pulmonary edema | Frothy, pink sputum; cough; bibasilar rales; S3 and S4; breathlessness; increased heart rate; decreased blood pressure | Exercise<br>Ventricular ischemia | Coronary artery disease<br>Mitral valve dysfunction<br>Outflow tract obstruction |

same site if it does recur? Is edema accompanied by a change in skin color or by pain, or is it pitting in nature? How does the patient gain relief from the edema or accompanying symptom of pain? Does he put his limb up? Does he wrap it with a counterpressure bandage? Does he use ice or heat? Does he take certain medications either to relieve it or to bring it on? What is the nature of associated complaints? For example, does the patient complain of wheezing? Of chest pain? Of local joint pain? What is the pain like?

What is the mental status of the patient?

### Implications for Physical Therapy

If edema has a cardiac etiology, monitor the electrocardiogram (ECG) during activity; if edema has a peripheral origin try to treat the cause.

## Physical Examination

### Physical Appearance

Patients with edema of cardiac origin show hallmark signs of right ventricular failure. They would have dependent, bilateral edema, and look cyanotic, with blue lips. They may appear obese, perhaps owing to ascites. Check for neck vein distention. When the patient lies recumbent at a 45° angle, are the neck veins at all prominent (filled with blood)? This is a clear indication of right ventricular failure.

Noncardiac etiologies for edema vary. Lymphedema is localized to one limb, but all other body parts should be normal in size, color, temperature, and skin appearance. Venous origins may present dependent bilateral edema, but there should be no jugular venous distension (JVD) and no cyanosis of lips or other appendages. There may be varicosities and skin discoloration with venous stasis. Arterial origins of edema are unusual but may include capillary bed inflammation or vasculitis. This is very painful, can quickly deteriorate to open lesions, which will not heal, and can occur anywhere.

### Vital Signs

As previously indicated, tachycardia may be a sign of heart failure accompanied by hypotension, and so heart rate and blood pressure should be measured. Respiratory rate and breath sounds help to determine the presence of left-sided heart failure, whereas bilateral ankle edema and hepatic enlargement or ascites may accompany right-sided heart failure. Heart sounds may be auscultated with the bell and diaphragm of the stethoscope placed on the apex of the heart. The audible S3 sound occurs in the presence of congestive heart failure (CHF) during early diastole, when there is an excessive amount of blood filling the ventricular chambers; this creates additional turbulence which results in greater than normal low-frequency noise.

## Tests

### Chest x-Ray

Cardiomegaly, or the "boot-shaped heart," and pulmonary edema may be seen, the latter as a "white out" of air spaces that should normally be black.

### Venography

Injection of contrast medium into large peripheral veins at their more distal points will permit x-ray pictures to show their size, their alignment, their tortuosity, and the integrity of venous valves.

### Lymphography

Large lymph channels can also be injected so that contrast pictures can show their function and integrity. Blockages cause massive edema and are usually due to tumor.

### Implications for Physical Therapy

Any treatment, such as heat, that relies upon normal blood flow to dissipate the extent of edema, should be reconsidered if there is a circulatory deficit. Heat is contraindicated in cases of arterial insufficiency.

## MEDICAL-SURGICAL INTERVENTION

Pharmacologic intervention for edema obviously depends upon the etiology and the severity of the problem. Once these have been ascertained, the drugs of choice are decided upon or surgery may be determined to be the only answer.

## Pharmacology

In CHF diuretics are used to reduce fluid load by reducing the circulating blood volume. Because ventricular function is poor, digitalis in one form or another may also be used because of its benefit in enhancing contractility of cardiac muscle. For inflammatory swelling, nonsteroidal anti-inflammatory agents, such as aspirin or Pyramidon, may be chosen.

## Invasive Monitoring

In some very sick patients with CHF central lines may be used for invasive monitoring. The Swan-Ganz catheter is threaded to the right ventricle and into the pulmonary artery, where the tip is wedged into the smaller-sized pulmonary arterial tree. A pressure transducer on the tip will then measure the pulmonary capillary wedge pressure which is an accurate indication of pulmonary hypertension in the case of pulmonary edema. For other arterial central lines see Chapter 4.

## Invasive Procedures

Surgical procedures may be indicated, especially in cases of lymphedema, when a clear tumor or obstruction is causing the massive swelling and fluid accumulation due to loss of a lymph outflow tract. Removal of tumor is very effective and apparently not detrimental to later function of a limb.

When CHF is present, the cause must be discovered. In the case of mitral valve dysfunction replacement of the valve with a porcine prosthesis or a synthetic metal prosthesis has relieved the problem. People with aortic valve dysfunction may suddenly develop fulminating pulmonary edema and need emergency valve replacement. To date, porcine valves seem to have the most success in terms of valve longevity.

When CHF cannot be compensated by the full battery of pharmacologic support, including experimental drugs, a patient may be considered a candidate for cardiac transplant surgery. Then a donor heart must be identified that is matched with respect to blood type and tissue type and is available within a few hours of death of the donor. Many transplant recipients have lived long years and found amazing levels of physical functioning (one such patient ran a marathon and continues to do so some years later).

## Physical Therapy Intervention

## Interview

In the initial interview the patient's answers to the general questions found in Chapter 3 may elucidate information already ascertained in chart review. Below are some additional key questions specific to the problem of edema, which may help the decision about the most appropriate treatment for the problem.

Add these key questions to generic physical therapy patient interview.

1. If you suspect CHF: Have you experienced weight gain recently? Has it been a sudden gain in the last 2 to 4 days? Are your ankles unusually

puffy? Do you have trouble breathing when you lie down flat? What brings on breathlessness?

2. If you suspect venous stasis: Do you have pain in your swollen leg? At rest? When you walk?

3. If you suspect trauma: Have you had any accidents or injuries recently? What medications do you take?

## Evaluation

In the physical therapy evaluation, include range of motion of edematous parts, general strength in affected limbs, balance and coordination, signs of recent or old trauma at the edematous site, chest evaluation if CHF is suspected (see Ch. 4) and vital signs (heart rate, respiratory rate, ECG rhythm, and breath sounds, heart sounds) where CHF may be implicated. Postural evaluation may be helpful, especially in cases of massive edema. Skin color in the area of edema will help determine vascular involvement, and girth measurement in the edematous region is useful, especially as a baseline objective measure for future comparison when treatment must be evaluated for its effectiveness. More sophisticated than girth measurement for the same purpose is volumetric measurement, done with special equipment for limb immersion. Venous occlusion plethysmography may be useful in some cases for measurement of limb blood flow (see Ch. 11). Most important from the physical therapy standpoint is a functional assessment, such as gait analysis if a lower extremity is edematous or some upper extremity function if the arm is involved. Thus the impairment from the edema may be judged, and treatment goals may be more appropriately assigned.

## Rehabilitation

Primarily, the first goal in rehabilitation is to remove excess fluid in the region of edema, if it impairs function, either through loss of range of motion (ROM), loss of muscular strength, or loss of coordination or by causing pain. Pain may be due to inflammation, to pressure, or to ischemia. If it is not cardiopulmonary in origin, then treatments are determined on the basis of the underlying cause and may include the use of thermal agents to reduce inflammation, physical treatments such as massage to enhance venous and lymphatic flow, or counterpressure devices such as a Jobst boot or elastic counterpressure bandage. Exercise to assist in venous return and internal massage may be beneficial. If pain is a limitation to exercise, pain relief may be sought before further rehabilitation may progress.

Edema from congestive heart failure is not reversed by exercise or any particular physical therapy modality. Diuresis is effective and takes some time. The patient who has uncompensated CHF should not exercise and may show ventricular ectopic activity as a consequence of the ventricular dysfunction.

# SUGGESTED READING

Ganong W: Review of Medical Physiology. 8th Ed. Lange Medical Books, Los Altos, CA, 1977

Stick C, Stüfen P, Witzleb E: On physiological edema in man's lower extremity. Eur J Appl Physiol 54:442, 1985

# CASE PROFILES

## Case 1: Diabetes Patient with Amputation and Chest Pain, Breathlessness, Irregular Heart Beat, and Leg Pain (Mr. P.)

Mr. P. is a 52-year-old diabetic below-knee amputee who is married, works as a history teacher in the local high school, and lives with his wife, two teenage sons, and ten-year-old daughter.

### MEDICAL HISTORY AND RISK FACTOR ASSESSMENT

No known history of cardiac disease. Multiple risk factors include:

Having diabetes mellitus for 20 years
Having hypertension, treated with hydrochlorothiazide, for 10 years
Four pack year smoking history (2 packs per day × 2 years), quit 20 years ago
Family history, includes father having MI at 50 years old, is now 76; mother has diabetes
Cholesterol value of 280 mg/dl 2 years prior to this admission

Table 1. Mr. P.'s Chronology of Medical Events

| Findings | Emergency room, Admission | Emergency Room, After Rx | Catheterization Laboratory | Coronary Care Unit, 8 hours After Admission |
|---|---|---|---|---|
| Vital signs | | | | |
| Heart rate (bpm) | 116 | 126 | 116 | Sinus tachycardia Ventricular ectopy |
| Blood pressure (mmHg) | 150/100 | 86/50 | – | 96/60 |
| Pulmonary capillary wedge (mmHg) | – | – | 34 | 15 |
| Respiratory rate (bpm) | 28 | 20 | 20 | 15 |
| Auscultation | | | | |
| Heart sounds | S3, S4 gallop | S3, S4 | – | S4 |
| Breath sounds | Rales, bilateral bases | Rales, bilateral bases | – | – |
| Laboratory values | | | | |
| ABG | Room air 75/40/7.34 | Room air 102/40/7.42 | 2 L nasal O$_2$ 104/40/7.4 | – |
| CPK U/ml | 200 | – | – | 1200 |
| MB band | too low | – | – | 21% |
| LDH U/ml | 30 | – | – | 335 |
| PTT seconds | 35.3 | – | – | 80 |
| Hematocrit | 44% | – | – | 43% |
| Hemoglobin gm/100 ml | 15 | – | – | 14 |
| Red blood cells million/mm$^3$ | 4.9 | – | – | 4.8 |

| | | | |
|---|---|---|---|
| Blood glucose mg/dl | 202 | — | — | 240 |
| Hemoglobin A 1 c | 6.2% | — | — | 6.2% |
| Cholesterol mg/dl | 220 | — | — | — |
| Triglycerides mg/dl | 306 | — | — | — |
| Electrocardiogram | ST ↑ V 1-6, Poor R wave progression V 1-6, rare PVC | Same | Same | Same |
| Chest x-ray | "White-out" lower lobes | — | — | Clear fields, IABP in position |
| Measurements of LV function | | | | |
| LV ejection fraction | — | — | 24% | 30% by echocardiogram, dilated LV |
| Cardiac output | — | — | 2.4 L/min | — |
| Wall motion | — | — | Antero-septal and anterolateral hypokinesis | Anteroseptal akinesis Anterior and anterolateral hypokinesis (by echocardiogram) |
| Medications | None | Oxygen SL nitroglycerine IV streptokinase Lasix | Same | IV nitroglycerine Heparin Digitalis Insulin Xanax |

Peripheral Vascular Disease (PVD) with recent left B/K amputation
Sedentary life style
Some stress experienced at home

# CHRONOLOGY OF MEDICAL EVENTS

Mr. P. is receiving gait training with a new prosthesis using parallel bars. He rapidly becomes unusually breathless, diaphoretic, and slightly nauseous. He sits down and decides to eat a hard candy, assuming that he is having a hypoglycemic reaction to exercise and his recent insulin injection. After a few minutes, Mr. P. states that he feels better, and convinces the therapist not to call the doctor. The therapist sends him home without working further in the parallel bars.

During the night, Mr. P. is brought to the Emergency Room (ER) by ambulance after 1½ hours of breathlessness, diaphoresis, and nausea.

He is given nitroglycerine, oxygen, IV lasix, and IV streptokinase. He is taken to the catheterization laboratory for evaluation of coronary artery disease (CAD) and possible therapeutic intervention including percutaneous transluminal coronary angioplasty (PTCA). Angiography reveals the following:

LAD: tight proximal lesion with 20 percent residual after PTCA
LCx: 80 percent stenosis proximal to first marginal with 0 percent residual after PTCA
RCA: small, irregular, without plaque

Mr. P. is taken to the coronary care unit (CCU) for monitoring and IABP support. Four hours after CCU admission Mr. P. is noted to be in ventricular bigeminy with several couplets. A bolus of lidocaine is administered with prompt suppression of dysrhythmia.

Table 1 summarizes the physical exam, test findings, and medical-surgical interventions from admission on through the CCU stay.

## Interpretation of Medical Events

The following list interprets the values and findings of Table 1.

1. Since this is a diabetic patient, the symptoms of breathlessness, and diaphoresis experienced during physical therapy were probably an anginal equivalent, especially since the patient went on to infarct. He showed classic denial of cardiac symptoms and talked his physical therapist out of more aggressive action (See Chs. 4, 5, and 8.)
2. ER events: What's going on here?

ECG findings suggest large area of the myocardium is in jeopardy.

Chest x-ray suggests congestive heart failure (CHF).

Blood gases show hypoxia.

Heart sounds are consistent with heart failure.

Breathlessness is consistent with heart failure.

Response to ER intervention is hypotension. Why?

Diuresis has decreased preload.

Nitroglycerine has decreased afterload and preload.

Large myocardial infarction (MI) has decreased contractility and force of contraction.

These three precipitate cardiogenic shock in Mr. P.

3. Catheterization lab report: What's going on here?

Mr. P. is still in CHF.

Hemodynamic measurements verify the clinical impression of cardiogenic shock.

Streptokinase may have opened up plaque in coronary vessels to some degree, permitting better blood flow to the myocardium.

PTCA should diminish the size of the lesions and the amount of myocardial necrosis. He has a very poor ejection fraction (EF).

4. CCU: What's going on here?

Akinesis in the anteroseptal wall suggests infarction with minimal salvage in the LAD supply territory.

Hypokinesis in the anterolateral wall suggests less injury, with possible salvage of the partial LCx supply territory.

IABP placed to rest the heart, perfuse coronary vessels, and thus allow recovery of the myocardium.

Bigeminy and couplets may either be a response to reperfusion of a portion of ventricle wall, or ventricular irritability typically found in the peri-infarction period.

His echocardiogram shows slight improvement of his EF.

# CHRONOLOGY OF EVENTS OCCURRING DURING HOSPITAL STAY

Mr. P. was weaned from his IABP after two days and his IV TNG was discontinued but replaced by sliding scale Isordil. Eight hours after removal of the IABP, his pulmonary capillary wedge (PCW) increased and Lasix was given, which brought it back to normal range. Occasional ventricular ectopic beats were noted unrelated to exertion. Resting sinus tachycardia persisted.

Mr. P. was transferred to the step down unit (SDU) on day 3 for telemetric monitoring, initiation of rehabilitation, and further tests.

In the SDU, Mr. P.'s heart rates ranged from 96 to 120 during his 5 days there. He also had occasional ectopy. On day 4 he was administered atenolol but developed shortness of breath, wheezing, and bibasilar rales after a test dose. His blood pressure remained stable at 100/60. By day 5 post-MI Mr. P. had his functional evaluation by the physical therapist.

Day 8 was his first day out of the SDU on the ward. He carried out his progressive rehabilitation activities throughout the next four days until discharge to home on day 12.

Table 2 shows events during Mr. P.'s stay in the SDU and on the hospital floor.

## Intrepretation of Hospital Events

The following list interprets the events which occurred during Mr. P.'s hospital stay.

1.  Events at 8 hours post IABP removal. What's going on here?

    Mr. P. had a sudden CHF decompensation, rectified by Lasix

    Ventricular ectopic activity (VEA) due to a highly irritable ventricle in the early stages of healing

    Sinus tachycardia is a mechanism to maintain his cardiac output since the ejection fraction remains quite low. This is a poor prognostic sign for Mr. P.

2.  SDU events; What's going on here?

    Atenolol was given to control his tachycardia and suppress ectopy. It was poorly tolerated because of poor ventricular function, tenuous CHF, and stunned myocardium. It was withdrawn.

    Groin hematoma from insertion of IABP and use of streptokinase. Be concerned about hematoma due to poor vessels and healing delay from diabetes.

3.  Events on hospital ward; What's going on here?

    New LVEF at 44 percent shows much improved ventricular function. This was primarily due to successful early reperfusion of ischemic regions, including the LCx territory as indicated by resolution of anterolateral hypokinesis seen on GBPS.

    Persantine thallium results reconfirm the extent of permanent damage and the presence of some ventricular dysfunction. Exercise thallium was not done because of his BK amputation.

    Atenolol is brought on board and is well tolerated now, due to improved ventricular function as confirmed by GBPS. Diltiazem protects myocardium from ischemia due to coronary vessel spasm.

    Persantine is a mild anticoagulant, necessary in post-PTCA.

    The ECG shows evolution of Q waves in the anteroseptal leads, indicating a transmural MI in this region of the heart.

**Table 2. Chronology of Hospital Events (Mr. P.)**

| Event | Step Down Unit | Floor |
|---|---|---|
| Length of stay | 5 days (Days 3–8) | 4 days (Days 9–12) |
| Vital signs | HR: 96–120, occasional VEA<br>BP: 100/60 | Days 8–10<br>HR: 96–110<br>BP: 110–120/82<br>RR: 15<br>Days 10–12<br>HR: 72–105<br>BP: 100–120/70 |
| Tests and evaluations | Large groin hematoma | Day 10: Gated Blood Pool Study: anteroseptal akinesis, LVEF = 44%<br>Day 11: Persantine Thallium reproduced chest pain, reversed with aminophylin, thallium showed fixed anteroseptal deficit, minimal redistribution anterior wall, minimum lung uptake |
| Electrocardiogram | Q waves in V1–V4 | Same |
| Medications | Day 4: test dose of atenolol; discontinued due to shortness of breath<br>Digitalis<br>Insulin<br>Heparin<br>Isordil | Day 10:  Atenolol<br>Diltiazem<br>Insulin<br>Persantine<br>Isordil |
| Rehabilitation | Day 5: interview and functional evaluation activity: transfers, independent self-care, ADL (see Table 3)<br><br>Education re: pulse, energy conservation technique, evaluation for prosthesis<br>Involve family in care and education<br>Description of activities for remainder of hospital stay | Days 6–12: walking with walker, stationary bicycling, ADL to include shower, stairs (see Table 4)<br>RPE: 11–12<br>Discharge evaluation (see Table 5)<br>Home program instruction |

## Initial Functional Evaluation of the Patient

Table 3 summarizes the first physical therapy functional evaluation performed on Day 5 in the SDU. All clinical findings are within normal limits; therefore, fatigue and breathlessness are primarily due to bedrest and extent of acute complications.

## Rehabilitation of the Patient During his Stay on the Hospital Floor

Table 4 lists the chronology of Mr. P.'s rehabilitation activities on days 6 through 11 of his hospital stay. All responses are within normal limits. Energy cost of ambulation with B/K prosthesis and walker is higher than energy cost of normal walking at same speed. However, walking with prosthesis is closer to normal range than swing-through gait using a walker without prosthesis.

## Discharge Functional Evaluation

Table 5 illustrates the clinical findings of the final functional evaluation before discharge from the hospital. All responses are within normal limits, but now resting and exercise values are lower due to change of medications; atenolol is a beta-blocker. Teach patients to avoid those forms of activity which pose a static load or Valsalva maneuver on the system. Both increase

---

**Table 3. Mr. P's. Functional Evaluation (SDU)**

Activities
  Supine → sit → stand
  Prosthesis donning
  Sit to bilateral stand on prosthesis
  Ambulation 15 feet with walker, bed to bathroom

Clinical Findings
  Heart rate:        102–120, no VEA
  Blood pressure:   100/60, 10 mmHg increase with activities
  Auscultation
    Heart sounds:    S4 present before and after activities
    Breath sounds:   Rales, cleared with deep inspiration and cough
  Symptoms:       Fatigue, breathlessness

Instructions
  Walk two times, each time for a length of 15 feet.
  Monitor pulse for irregular heart beat and heart rate.
  Pace all activities throughout day.
  Practice energy conservation techniques.

**Table 4. Chronology of Rehabilitation During Hospital Stay (Mr. P.)**

| Day | Activity[a] | Responses |
|-----|-------------|-----------|
| 6 | Walk with walker 3 minutes with PT with prosthesis and one rest | HR: 96–105<br>BP: 110/80–120/82<br>No change in heart or lung sound<br>RR: 15 |
| 7 | Walker ambulation 3 minutes with PT<br>Walker ambulation 3 minutes independently, 3 times | HR: 96–98 (by PT)<br>HR: 98–110 (by patient) |
| 8 & 9 | Walks daily 3–5 min with walker, 5 times<br>Sit-down shower | Keep HR below 110 |
| 10 & 11 | Walk 5–10 min with PT, self–monitoring pulse<br>Stationary bicycling with PT, 5–10 min | Keep HR below 110<br>RPE 11 |

[a] Walking sessions include prosthetic gait training.

**Table 5. Mr. P.'s Functional Physical Therapy Evaluation at Discharge**

Activities
  10 minute walk with prosthesis and walker
  10 minute stationary bicycle, free wheel
  Down and up one flight of stairs with prosthesis and hand rail

Clinical Findings
  Heart rate:        70 → 90, no VEA
  Blood pressure:    100/70 → 120/76
  RPP (max):         10,800
  RPE:               12
  Auscultation
    Heart sounds:    No change
    Breath sounds:   No change
  Symptoms:          Breathlessness, leg fatigue
  Medications:       Atenolol
                     Diltiazem
                     Insulin
                     Persantine
                     Isordil

Instructions
  One flight of stairs limited to RPE 12 and HR 90.
  Other activities not exceeding RPE 12 and HR 90, eg: gardening, riding stationary bike, walking up and down slight slopes, curbs; resume sexual activity with usual partner.
  Avoid isometric holding contractions; avoid breath-holding.
  Add 5 minutes to each modality every two days, limiting RPE and HR as above.
  Return in 3 weeks for re-evaluation and activity progression.

intrathoracic pressure and generate a high pressor response, thus increasing afterload.

## LONG TERM REHABILITATION

Mr. P. goes home, follows instructions, and returns after 3 weeks, when he reports doing the following activities: driving, raking, gardening, dining out occasionally, and going to church. He begins to practice his golf swing. He states he wants to try some new activities: playing golf, washing the car, going back to work, and finishing the deck on his house.

Mr. P. reports that for exercise he has walked 45 minutes with his prosthesis and walker once. He has biked 30 minutes without symptoms. His maximum HR has been 90, with an RPE of 10. He walks at a 50 step per minute pace, and bikes at 50 to 60 RPM freewheeling.

### The Three-week Outpatient Physical Therapy Visit

Table 6 illustrates the results of the clinical evaluation at the three-week outpatient physical therapy visit.

#### Interpretation of the Three-week Clinical Evaluation

All responses are within normal limits.

Our decision to let him play golf for 45 minutes is based on his safe performance under our supervision and his asymptomatic walking for that duration.

Our decision to let him wash his car only after safe performance of arm exercise with 5-pound weights is based on clinical judgment of his responses and of how strenuous car washing activity is.

Mr. P.'s question on return to work is not usually the domain of the physical therapist.

Our decision to deny him his request to work on his deck is based on our judgment of how much arm work is involved, both dynamic and static.

He needs to check blood sugars before and after exercise, since his insulin requirements may alter as his exercise increases.

### Six-week Outpatient Physical Therapy Visit (Exercise Tolerance Test)

Table 7 illustrates the results of the clinical evaluation at the 6-week outpatient visit, during which an exercise tolerance test (ETT) was done.

**Table 6. Mr. P.'s 3-Week Outpatient Visit: Functional Physical Therapy Evaluation**

Activities
    Warm up stretches
    Stationary bicycle 5 minutes, 25 watts
    Walk with prosthesis and one cane instruction, 10 minutes at 50 spm
    Golf swing with golf club

Clinical Findings

| | |
|---|---|
| Heart rate: | $70 \rightarrow 100$, no pauses in pulse |
| Blood pressure: | $100/70 \rightarrow 125/80$ |
| RPP: | 12,500 |
| RPE: | 13 |
| Auscultation | |
|   Heart sounds: | Normal |
|   Breath sounds: | Clear |
| Symptoms: | None |
| Medications: | Atenolol |
| | Diltiazem |
| | Insulin |
| | Persantine |
| | Isordil |

Instructions
    Walk 45 minutes a day, limiting RPE to 13 and HR to 100; after remaining within these limits for one week, he may golf one time per week.
    Begin upper extremity exercise to include 2 pound weights in each hand using functional diagonal patterns, 10 repetitions once per day, building up to 3 sets of 10 repetitions, staying within prescribed RPE 13. Once Mr. P. achieves 3 sets of 10 repetitions with 5 pound weights, he may wash his car.
    Mr. P. should discuss his return to work with his doctor. He could begin preparing lectures and handouts, while still at home.
    He should not begin work on his deck.
    Progress to 60 spm walk with cane and prosthesis for 45 minutes daily
    Ride stationary bike at 50 to 60 repetitions per minute (RPM), beginning with 5 minutes free-wheeling, each time, and ending with a 5 minute cool down each time, spending: 5 minutes at 25 watts daily for first week; 10 minutes at 25 watts daily for second week; 15 minutes at 25 watts daily for third week.
    Continue to check blood sugar for insulin requirement.
    Return in 3 weeks for scheduled bike ETT.

## Interpretation of Six-week Evaluation

Mr. P.'s lipid values are too high and present a moderate risk for recurrent MI. Therefore a dietary or medical program should be initiated.

The intensity of exercise for his training prescription is 70 to 85 percent of the maximum HR achieved on the ETT. This is required for an aerobic conditioning effect. As a fairly young diabetic, a more frequent, longer duration of exercise should help to normalize his glucose metabolism.

The decision to enroll patients in supervised cardiac rehabilitation programs may be based on several factors including:

1. Financial status
2. Distance for patient to travel

Table 7. Mr. P.'s 6-Week Outpatient Physical Therapy Visit (ETT)

Activity
  Stationary bicycle ergometer with prosthesis
    Continous protocol with 25 watt increments every 3 minutes
    Stopped in 10.5 minutes at 100 watts

Clinical Findings
  Heart rate:           75 → 130
  ECG:                  negative for ischemia, angina; occasional PACs during and after
                          exercise
  Blood pressure:       100/70 → 150/88
  RPP:                  19,500
  RPE:                  19
  Auscultation
    Heart sounds:       S4 after exercise
    Breath sounds:      Normal
  Symptoms:             None, stopped due to leg fatigue
  Medications:          Unchanged from 3 week evaluation
  Total cholesterol:    240 mg/dl
  Triglycerides         105 mg/dl
  LDL:                  179 mg/dl
  HDL:                  40 mg/dl
  Total cholesterol/
    HDL:                6.0
  Potassium:            4.2 mEq/L
  Blood glucose:        98 mg/dl    .

Instructions
  Begin the phase 3 cardiac rehabilitation program, independent or supervised setting.
  Exercise prescription
    Frequency: 5 days per week
    Duration: 60 minutes total (split between modalities)
    Modality: walking, cycling, and upper body aerobic exercise
    Intensity: (70–85%) × 130 = 91 to 110 beats per minute
  Dietary modifications: Reduction in total cholesterol and LDL to improve ratio closer to
    4.0, reduction in triglyceride
  Re-evaluation stress test and labs in 12 weeks.
  Discuss return to work with physician.

3.  Compliance with exercise prescription
4.  Medical stability

Mr. P. has done extremely well and is apparently stable and compliant. He also shows good judgment and so could carry on independently. After Mr. P.'s doctor sees this excellent stress test result, he tells Mr. P. to return to his job. His doctor will see him again in 6 months.

# SUGGESTED READINGS

APTA Anthology: Energy Cost: Studies Related to Physical Therapy. American Physical Therapy Association, Alexandria, Virginia, 1981

Amsterdam E, Wilmore J, DeMaria A: Exercise in Cardiovascular Health and Disease. Yorke Medical Books, New York, 1977

Irwin S, Tecklin J: Cardiopulmonary Physical Therapy. CV Mosby, St. Louis, 1985
Pollock, M, Schmidt D (ed): Heart Disease and Rehabilitation. Houghton-Mifflin, Boston, 1979
Wenger N (ed): Exercise and the Heart. Cardiovascular Clinics. 2nd Ed. FA Davis, Philadelphia, 1985

# Case 2: Chronic Obstructive Pulmonary Disease (COPD) Patient with Breathlessness, Cough, Leg Pain, Irregular Heart Beat, Fatigue, Lightheadedness, Loss of Consciousness (Mr. F.)

Mr. F. is a 58-year-old-male who is scheduled for a right total hip replacement in 4 weeks. He is referred to physical therapy as an outpatient for a conditioning program prior to surgery.

## MEDICAL HISTORY AND RISK FACTOR ASSESSMENT

His medical history includes bilateral lower extremity peripheral neuropathy, and he had a fall because of this problem. As a result of his fall 6 years ago, he fractured his right femoral neck and has had recurrent hip pain consistent with degenerative joint disease. He also has right calf pain with ambulation. He was a heavy smoker for 30 years and has emphysema with a chronic dry cough. He breathes with accessory muscles and is barrel-chested.

Table 8 lists information gleaned from the review of his medical chart.

### Interpretation of Medical Chart Review

1. Pulmonary function tests show that Mr. F. has severe emphysema, with both a restrictive and obstructive component.
2. ECG and chest x-ray, auscultatory findings, and echocardiogram (ECHO) all indicate that the right atrium of his heart is enlarged. This happens with severe obstructive lung disease over a period of many years. His tubular lung sounds are consistent with the appearance of blebs on his chest x-ray, and his diagnosis of panlobular emphysema.

**Table 8. Mr. F.'s Medical Chart Review**

| | |
|---|---|
| Physical examination | Height: 67 inches<br>Weight: 129 lb<br>Remarkable for enlarged prostate |
| Auscultation | Heart sounds: widening of physiologic split in S2<br>Breath sounds: tubular |
| Cough | Nonproductive |
| Lab Values | ABGs: normal    labs: normal |
| Pulmonary function tests | observed  predicted  percent<br>VC   2.05    4.37    48<br>$FEV_1$  1.79    3.45    52<br>RV   3.14    2.24   140 |
| Electrocardiogram | Right atrial hypertrophy (increased P in V1); PACs; non-specific ST-T wave changes; right bundle branch block |
| Chest x-ray | Panlobular emphysematous blebs |
| Echocardiogram | Right atrial hypertrophy |
| Lower extremity arteriography | Right internal iliac artery disease at bifurcation: right blood flow decreased greater than left |
| Social history | Disabled due to lung disease; previously a janitor |
| Medicines | Theodur; Ventolin; Trental |

3. Arteriography shows low flows in the iliac artery which are consistent with his calf pain symptom of intermittent claudication.

# FIRST PHYSICAL THERAPY VISIT

Mr. F. is seen in physical therapy for the initial evaluation and interview. He is very motivated to comply with our plans and can come to the hospital daily if necessary. He drives and gets around independently. He lives with his wife who works full-time in a bank. Their two children are grown and self-supporting. Mr. F. lives in an apartment building with an elevator and has access to his neighbor's stationary bike.

Table 9 lists the results of Mr. F.'s initial physical therapy evaluation.

## Interpretation of Initial Physical Therapy Evaluation

1. Chest assessment shows the typical pink puffer emphysema patient with stiff rib cage and very poor posture which interferes with diaphragmatic function. Postural re-alignment along with correction of paradoxical

**Table 9. Mr. F.'s Initial Physical Therapy Evaluation**

Activities
  Chest assessment (See Ch. 3, generic cardiopulmonary evaluation)
  Musculoskeletal evaluation: ROM and MMT of both lower extremities
  Functional and endurance evaluations:
    6 minute walk test, walking with cane in left hand; claudication in RLE began after 3
      minutes of walking; he slowed his pace until completion; he completed 1,000 feet in 6
      minutes, limited by leg pain and breathlessness.
    UBE (Cybex Isokinetic Upper Body Exerciser) setting at 120, at 60 RPM for 5 minutes.
    Stationary bicycle, freewheel, limited by R hip pain after 10 minutes

Clinical findings
  Musculoskeletal
    ROM: LLE: normal range and strength

| | |
|---|---|
| RLE: hip flexion: | 20–120 degrees |
| Hip extension: | –20 degrees |
| Hip internal rotation: | 10–15 degrees |
| Hip external rotation: | –10–0 degrees |
| Hip abduction: | 0–15 degrees |
| Hip adduction: | 0–30 degrees |
| MMT: RLE: hip: | Fair |
| Knee flexion: | Good |
| Knee extension, | Fair |

        with degrees limited by pain
      Endurance: fair
    Chest: Stiff rib cage; poor chest wall mobility

  Cardiopulmonary
    Inspection: Use of accessory muscles
              Shows paradoxical abdominal motion
              Both patterns increase with exercise
              Begins pursed lips breathing with exercise
              Postural deviations: hunched, elevated shoulders, kyphosis, foward head
              Posterior pelvic tilt
              Appears as "pink-puffer"
              Looks frail, thin
              Trophic skin changes over both ankles and feet
    Palpation: I:E (inspiratory to expiratory time ratio) 1:4
            Lacks right tibial and popliteal pulses
            Skin temperature cooler on right leg
    Percussion: Resonant sounds over all segments
    Auscultation
      Heart sounds: as per medical record; no change with exercise
      Breath sounds: tubular
    Vital signs

| | |
|---|---|
| Heart rate: | 120 → 96 bpm |
| Heart rhythm: | resting and exercise PACs 12–15/minute |
| Blood pressure: | 122/84 → 166/90 |
| Respiratory rate: | 16 → 20 |
| RPE: | 16 |
| RPP: | 14,640 → 15,936 |
| Symptoms: | Breathlessness |
| | Leg pain |
| | Irregular heart beat |
| | Cough |

Instructions
  Return 3× week to work on UBE, stationary bicycle, hip stretching and strengthening
    and breathing retraining.
  Follow independent walking endurance program as his hip and leg pain allow.
  Use stationary bicycle at home in same protocol as in the physical therapy department.

breathing pattern and facilitation of the diaphragm are all required. Chest wall mobilization and increased efficiency of use of muscles of breathing will help.

2. Functional impairment in walking is due to both his mechanical inefficiency of breathing with very high oxygen cost of breathing, as well as to combined musculoskeletal pain of malaligned hip and to claudication pain of the calf.

3. Mr. F. shows an elevated resting heart rate of 120 which drops to 96 when he walks, or does upper body exercise or stationary bicycling. This is a common finding in patients on methylxanthine sympathomimetic drugs. These medications act like adrenalin to cause tachycardia, but with exercise, their influence upon the sino-atrial node appears to be supplanted by the exercise demands for an adequate cardiac output, which is met by an elevation from the resting stroke volume value and a lower heart rate. We note an adaptive blood pressure response showing this alteration.

## PHYSICAL THERAPY PROGRAM

Mr. F. returns 3 times per week for therapy. He makes very little progress with his walking program because of his hip pain. His onset of claudication remains unchanged over the 4 weeks. Similarly, his right hip ROM remains unchanged. His right lower extremity (RLE) strength shows minimal improvement.

Table 10 shows Mr. F's exercise progression.

### Interpretation of Exercise Progression

Breathing retraining program emphasizes improvement of breathing pattern rather than other pulmonary hygiene because he has little to no sputum production, has near normal arterial blood gases (ABGs) (pure emphysema), and his major problem is a very high oxygen cost of breathing with a very inefficient musculoskeletal pump. Over 4 weeks he learns to control diaphragm descent voluntarily with a looser abdominal wall, and to rely less on accessory muscles for inspiration, at rest, and beginning to develop his coordination with activity.

Both UBE and cycle exercise show the elevated heart rate at rest, with the drop with exercise. As a training effect appears, the higher exercising heart rates are possible due to the increase in duration of work performed, or increase in intensity of work. Now the demand for cardiac output is sufficiently high to raise HR above resting tachycardia of 120 produced by the methylxanthine medication.

UBE cardiac responses are higher than leg cycling due to the expected differences of arm work vs. leg work.

**Table 10. Chronology of Exercise (Mr. F.)**

| Intervention | Week 1 | Week 2 | Week 3 | Week 4 |
|---|---|---|---|---|
| Breathing retraining | Tolerated 5 minutes supine with anterior pelvic tilt using diaphragmatic breathing (passive prolonged stretch to tight abdominal muscles) | Tolerated 10 minutes supine with ant. pelvic tilt using diaphragmatic breathing. Quick stretch to diaphragm at initiation of inspiration added to program and tolerated | Tolerating ant. pelvic tilt and use of diaphragmatic breathing in sitting and standing | Incorporates ant. pelvic tilt and diaphragmatic breathing while walking and using UBE with PT coaching |

Endurance training program
UBE 60 rpm

| | Week 1 | Week 2 | Week 3 | Week 4 |
|---|---|---|---|---|
| Duration: | 5 minutes | 10 minutes | 12 minutes | 15 minutes |
| HR: | 120–100 | 120–105 | 120–110 | 120–112 |
| Rhythm: | PACs, 12–15/min | PACs, 12–15/min | PACs 10–12/min | PACs 10–12/min |
| BP: | 122/84–150/86 | 120/84–150/82 | 116/80–146/82 | 116/78–142/80 |
| RR: | 16–20 | 16–20 | 16–20 | 16–20 |
| RPE: | 16 | 15 | 14 | 14 |
| Symptoms: | Breathlessness, arm fatigue | Breathlessness, arm fatigue | Breathlessness, arm fatigue | Breathlessness, arm fatigue |

Stationary bicycling freewheel

| | Week 1 | Week 2 | Week 3 | Week 4 |
|---|---|---|---|---|
| Duration: | 10 min continuous | 10 minutes work<br>5 minutes rest<br>10 minutes work | 15 minutes work<br>3 minutes rest<br>10 minutes work | 15 minutes work<br>3 minutes rest<br>15 minutes work |
| HR: | 120–96 | 120–102 | 120–110 | 120–124 |
| Rhythm: | PACs | PACs | PACs | PACs |
| BP: | 122/84–136/84 | 120/84–140/84 | 116/80–130/82 | 116/78–128/80 |
| RR: | 16–19 | 16–19 | 16–19 | 16–18 |
| RPE: | 15 | 14 | 14 | 13 |
| Symptoms: | Hip pain, leg fatigue, breathlessness | Hip pain, leg fatigue, breathlessness | Hip pain, leg fatigue, breathlessness | Hip pain, leg fatigue, breathlessness |

## POSTSURGICAL REHABILITATION

Mr. F. undergoes an uncomplicated total hip replacement and is referred back to physical therapy for progressive ambulation with crutches, ADL instruction, and breathing retraining. On day 2 postoperative, the therapist resumes the therapeutic program, including instructions regarding bed mobility and transfer to chair to increase sitting tolerance. After 5 minutes of dangling his legs at the bedside, Mr. F. is asked to stand and pivot into the chair. Upon standing, Mr. F. says he feels dizzy and becomes diaphoretic, and his knees buckle. The therapist is able to place him supine in bed and palpate a radial pulse as Mr. F. wakes, asking, "what happened?" After explaining to Mr. F. that he fainted and reassuring him that this was not uncommmon after a surgery such as his, the therapist measured his BP and HR. These were 110/80 and 126 and irregular. After waiting for 5 minutes, a repeat BP was taken, and another more gradual attempt to sit, dangle, and stand was made. Sitting, BP dropped to 104/80 and after 5 minutes, remained low at 100/80. He complained of some dizziness, but after sitting for 5 more minutes, doing ankle pumps, he no longer felt dizzy and his BP was stable. He was then able to stand and do a pivot transfer successfullly. His pulse remained irregular throughout, and was 136 when his systolic BP was 100.

## Interpretation of Medical Events: What's Going on Here?

Mr. F. has had an orthostatic hypotension response to change in position. With general anesthesia and the long surgical procedure, the responsiveness of peripheral vessel smooth muscles to baroreceptor stimulation to vasoconstrict is slower. The second time he tried sitting and standing there was some orthostatic intolerance but a compensatory tachycardia and the returning blood volume from his ankle pumps facilitated adequate perfusion to his brain. Irregular pulse continues and when monitored on ECG shows premature atrial contractions (PACs) as before.

## LONG-TERM REHABILITATION

Mr. F. begins to tolerate longer periods of sitting as his circulatory system adjusts. Later that same day, he demonstrates safe independent transfers. Over the next week he progresses to independent crutch ambulation with partial weight-bearing on level ground. He is sent home 1½ weeks after surgery but prior to discharge the therapist shows him stair climbing techniques with crutches and paced breathing. He is instructed to do all functional

Table 11. Mr. F.'s Discharge Functional Evaluation

Activities
  Chest assessment
  Walking 6 minutes with crutches, goes 2,000 feet, limited by breathlessness and left calf
    pain which comes on at 4.5 minutes
  UBE at 60 rpm (120 speed setting) for 10 minutes
  ROM, MMT, stationary bike deferred until R hip adequately healed

Clinical findings
  Chest assessment:    unchanged from pre-op
  Vital signs
    HR:               $126 \rightarrow 110$
    Rhythm:           resting and exercise 12–15 PACs/minute
    BP:               $116/82 \rightarrow 156/90$
    RR:               $16 \rightarrow 20$
    RPE:              17 peak
    RPP:              14,616 rest
                      17,160 peak
  Auscultation
    Heart sounds:     Unchanged from pre-op
    Breath sounds:    Unchanged from pre-op
  Medications:        Theodur
                      Ventolin
                      Trental
                      Persantine
  Symptoms:           Breathlessness
                      R hip incisional pain
                      L leg claudication
                      Irregular heart beat
                      Cough

Instructions
  Continue walking program increasing by time, keeping RPE at 13 to 15 and HR less than
    126. He should walk until left calf pain becomes too severe to continue, then rest, and
    resume walking when pain resolves. For a goal, he should try to achieve a total of one
    hour walking time each day, at first, partial weightbearing with crutches, and later, with
    his surgeon's approval, full weightbearing with crutches or with a cane.
  He should continue practicing his diaphragmatic breathing pattern and postural
    adjustments as he walks.
  He may resume a conditioning program on the stationary bicycle when his surgeon gives
    permission to resume this type of program.

activities at home, but to return in 1 week for continuation of his conditioning and breathing program.

Table 11 illustrates the clinical findings of the final functional evaluation before discharge.

## Interpretation of the Discharge Functional Evaluation: What's Going on Here?

Mr. F. experiences left calf claudication for the first time when he walks with crutches, bearing partial weight on the right for longer than a few minutes. We knew from arteriography that he had reduced flows to the left leg but remained asymptomatic as long as muscular demands were not as great. Now he is using more weight on the left leg, and partial weight on his right leg.

Crutch walking with partial weightbearing can have as much as a 25 percent increase in energy cost over normal walking. This form of walking therefore could be intense enough to provide a conditioning stimulus. Once he graduates to more normal walking, his right calf pain will most likely return. Stationary bicycling may be very helpful for functional improvement of claudication symptoms, as well as of cardiopulmonary conditioning.

Cardiopulmonary conditioning will help to reduce his breathlessness symptom perhaps by improving oxygen utilization in the periphery and thus creating lower oxygen demand on the emphysematic lungs. His paced breathing will help reduce the oxygen cost of moving air into and out of his lungs.

## SUGGESTED READING

Irwin S, Tecklin J: Cardiopulmonary Physical Therapy, CV Mosby, St Louis, 1985

# Case 3: Paraplegic Patient with Chest Pain, Breathlessness, Fatigue, and Cough (Mr. G.)

## MEDICAL HISTORY AND RISK ASSESSMENT

Mr. G. is a 72-year-old man who has been a paraplegic from poliomyelitis since 1938. He is ambulatory with bilateral Lofstrand crutches using a long leg brace on his right leg and a short leg brace on his left leg. He is seen as an outpatient in the physical therapy clinic for chronic low back pain which has recently become much worse, limiting his ability to walk to only 100 feet.

Mr. G. has a remote history of angina over several years, but has never been exercise-tested because of his physical disability. Mr. G. is overweight and sedentary since he ambulates infrequently due to back pain, but is independent in ADL. He lives one flight upstairs in an apartment with his wife who is a retired nurse. He smokes, and enjoys large meals and rich foods. He is a former printer who owned his own printing business. He has a strong family history for CAD, since both of his two brothers have had CABG surgery.

## CHRONOLOGY OF MEDICAL EVENTS

Upon walking from the parking lot (about 500 feet) for his fifth physical therapy treatment, he experiences fatigue, soreness of both elbows and wrists, shortness of breath, and is diaphoretic. He is convinced that he has some gastrointestinal (GI) distress, that his arms are hurting because he thinks he needs new crutches, and he slept poorly over the past few nights because his wife has a "bug," and his back has been particularly bad. He is confident that a rest, and his physical therapy treatment will make him feel better.

The physical therapist recognizes that Mr. G. may be denying symptoms

**240**

Table 12. Mr. G.'s Chronology of Medical Findings

| Measurement | PT Department | Emergency Room | Coronary Care Unit |
|---|---|---|---|
| Vital signs | | | |
| HR: | 110 bpm | Same | 66 bpm |
| Rhythm: | regular | Same | regular |
| BP: | 150/100 | 168/108 | 110/72 |
| RR: | 16 | 24 | 16 |
| Temperature: | 98.6°F | Same | Same |
| Auscultation | | | |
| Heart sounds: | Normal | Same | Same |
| Lung sounds: | Rhonchi, scattered rales | Same | Same |
| Lab Values | | | |
| Enzymes | | | |
| CPK: | – | 25 | 30 |
| LDH: | – | 62 | 60 |
| SGOT: | – | 40 | 42 |
| Lipids | | | |
| Cholesterol: | – | 320 | – |
| Triglycerides: | | 500 | – |
| Electrocardiogram | – | T wave inversion, leads 2,3, aVF | T waves normalize |
| Chest x-ray | – | Clear | Clear |
| Symptoms | Breathlessness Diaphoretic (atypical angina), chronic cough | Bilateral arm pain, chronic cough | Arm pain gone, cough persists |
| Medications | Sublingual nitroglycerine, Advil | 0.3 mg sublingual nitroglycerine ×3, IV morphine sulphate, 2 L O₂ via nasal prongs | Isordil Propranolol Advil |

of cardiovascular distress and decides to measure vital signs. Mr. G. has nitroglycerine tablets in his pocket but has not used them for over three years. Mr. G. takes one nitroglycerine tablet sublingually only after the therapist insists. After 5 minutes, he admits that bilateral arm pain persists but says he did not feel burning or tingling from the nitroglycerine on his tongue.

The therapist gets a wheelchair and notifies Mr. G.'s doctor that he is going to the emergency room. Mr. G. is admitted to the hospital coronary care unit to rule out the possibility of an acute MI. He is released from the hospital after 24 hours, and is scheduled for a persantine thallium test.

Table 12 lists the various medical findings recorded during the sequence of events which occurred.

## Interpretation of Medical Events

Patient shows strong denial of his confusing angina pectoris.

Nitroglycerine lasts 3 to 6 months. His was older, and weaker, as noted by lack of burning or tingling on his tongue.

He was admitted to the hospital even though the enzymes drawn in the ER were low, and there were minimal ECG changes. The physician was concerned that Mr. G.'s current symptom could deteriorate to unstable angina and infarction, especially in view of his previous history of angina and the fact that he now required large doses of medication to control his angina.

His medical regime of isordil and propranolol is one for typical angina control and works by limiting $M\dot{V}O_2$.

## POST-HOSPITALIZATION EVENTS

He is home for one day on isordil and propranolol, and experiences a recurrence of his arm pain. He calls his physician who schedules him for a cardiac catheterization within the next 2 weeks and cancels the persantine thallium test. The latter test is performed before catheterization to determine if one is necessary.

---

Catheterization report:
85 percent RCA stenosis
60 percent LCx stenosis
Catheter tip induces spasm of coronaries, reproduces his symptoms.
EF is 62 percent with normal wall motion
$\dot{Q}$ is 4.2 L/min
PCW = 18 mmHg
ECG: 2 mm ST segment depression in leads 2, 3, aVF, and chest pain during spasm

---

Conclusion: Medical management indicated. Add nifedipine to his medicines to control spasm. His catheterization report indicates one serious stenosis which does not compromise his ventricular function. After the catheterization his BP was 98/60, his HR was 62, and he was instructed to recommence physical therapy for his low back pain as well as to begin a risk factor modification program. This should include an aerobic training program when his back can tolerate it, smoking cessation, weight reduction, and dietary modifications.

## LONG TERM REHABILITATION

Mr. G. returns for low back pain therapy in 3 weeks and after 6 weeks of back exercises, successful weight reduction, and smoking cessation (1 week) he experiences much relief and is ready for aerobic exercise. An arm ergometry stress test is done.

Table 13 illustrates Mr. G.'s exercise tolerance test and lab results.

## Interpretation of ETT and Lab Results

The exercise test showed low physical working capacity, but hemodynamic responses were adaptive.

Wheezing could be bronchospasm due to COPD (smoking) and/or Inderal.

Myocardial ischemia on his ECG is consistent with his catheterization report.

Elbow/wrist pain is clearly his angina, and he needs to be able to recognize it.

His lipid levels indicate the possibility of a familial disorder, since weight loss brought cholesterol down by only 20 mg/dl. He probably needs lipid lowering medications, and should consult a dietician and/or endocrinologist.

The intensity, frequency, and duration are minimal for aerobic conditioning effects due to his tenuous low back pain situation and his age. To progress him, duration should be increased.

He is monitored once per week, not three times, to prevent the high energy cost of coming into therapy, but it is important to keep a close watch on his low back pain, his wheezing, his cough, and his angina.

## Functional Physical Therapy Evaluation

At his next visit to therapy, he is monitored during a functional walk (using braces and crutches) to see whether his responses fall within his target, or are excessive. If they are not excessive, this can be a useful exercise mode.

Table 14 lists the clinical findings of the functional physical therapy evaluation.

### Interpretation of the Functional Evaluation

The functional walk was more stressful to Mr. G.'s heart than the arm cranking test. This probably was due to two factors: he experienced local muscle fatigue at the arm cranking activity which limited his performance, and his walking activity with braces and crutches requires a higher energy cost than an arm cranking test.

Use of prophylactic TNG will lower the $M\dot{V}O_2$ and allow him to do

**Table 13. Mr. G.'s Exercise Test and Lab Results**

Activity
  Arm ergometry
  Intermittent protocol, 3 minutes work–3 minutes rest
    12.5 watts per stage
    Completed 37.5 watts

Clinical Findings
  Vital signs

| | |
|---|---|
| HR and rhythm: | 68 → 120 no VEA |
| BP: | 110/72 → 166/80 |
| RR: | 16 → 26 |
| RPP: | 19,920 peak |
| RPE: | 19 peak |

  Auscultation

| | |
|---|---|
| Heart sounds: | Normal |
| Breath sounds: | Expiratory wheeze upon completion of test |
| ECG | 1 mm horizontal ST depression in leads 2, 3, aVF at peak |
| Symptoms: | Breathlessness, elbow and wrist pain at peak, resolved with cessation of exercise test |
| | Test stopped for arm fatigue and wheeze |
| Medications: | Same as postcardiac catheterization |
| | isordil, propranolol, nifedipine, SL TNG, Advil |

  Lipids, fasting

| | |
|---|---|
| Total cholesterol: | 300 mg/dl |
| Triglycerides: | 460 mg/dl |
| HDL: | 28 mg/dl |
| LDL: | 180 mg/dl |
| Total Cholesterol/HDL: | 10 |

Instructions
  Aerobic exercise program
    Modality: arm cranking, swimming
    Frequency: 3 × per week, minimum
    Duration: 30 minutes
    Intensity: keep HR 84 to 102, keep RPE 13 to 15
  Dietary modifications
    Continue with low saturated fat and low cholesterol diet, recommend consultation with dietician, and recommend consultation with endocrinologist for consideration of cholesterol lowering drugs and evaluation of hypertriglyceridemia.
  Return one time each week for monitoring of walking and arm cranking program.
  Recommend strategies to continue cigarette avoidance.
  Notify therapist if he needs assistance in secretion removal or if he notices a change in color, quantity, consistency of sputum.
  Notify therapist of any exacerbation of low back pain.
  If elbow/wrist pain occurs, stop exercise and take SL TNG, and contact doctor if it persists, reoccurs more frequently, or requires more than 3 TNG for relief.

more overall work before he gets his angina. There is a possibility that his isordil should be increased if he needs SL TNG frequently.

The walking interval program is selected in order to prevent his heart from becoming ischemic. Interval training has been shown to be effective in providing a conditioning effect as long as the rest interval is shorter than the exercise interval.

**Table 14. Mr. G.'s Functional Physical Therapy Evaluation**

Activity
  Walking, 6 minutes with Lofstrand crutches and braces, 800 feet (long leg brace on right, short leg brace on left)

Clinical Findings
  Vital signs
    HR:         68 → 120 bpm
    BP:         110/72 → 180/80
    RPE:        16
    RPP:        21,600
    RR:         16 → 30
  Auscultation
    Heart sounds:  Normal
    Lung sounds:   Wheeze
  Symptoms:     Breathlessness, cough, elbow and wrist pain (received 0.3 mg SL TNG, with relief)
  Medications:  Isordil,
                Propranolol
                Nifedipine
                SL TNG
                Advil

Instructions
  If Mr. G. needs to walk longer than 5 minutes, he should take a prophylactic TNG.
  For walking exercise program, 3 to 5 minute intervals with 1 to 2 minute rest periods may prevent angina and protect from back pain.

# SUGGESTED READINGS

APTA Anthology: Energy Cost: Studies Related to Physical Therapy. American Physical Therapy Association, Alexandria, Virginia, 1981

Fisher S V, Gullickson G: Energy Cost of Ambulation of Health and Disability: A Literature Review. Arch Phys Med & Rehab 59:124, 1978

# Case 4: Geriatric Patient with Breathlessness, Cough, Fatigue, Irregular Heart Beat, and Edema (Pulmonary) (Mrs. S.)

Mrs. S. is a 77-year-old female with a history of alcoholism, chronic obesity, cigarette abuse, and rheumatic heart disease, with known mitral stenosis and recent appearance of mitral regurgitation by echocardiogram. She is currently admitted for right cerebrovascular accident (CVA). She has been receiving bedside physical therapy for 1 week and the therapist is considering initiating treatment in the department in order to utilize the mat and parallel bars and a larger area for wheelchair propulsion.

## MEDICAL HISTORY

Periodic physical exams in the past 10 years have revealed the following:

Ten years prior to admission (PTA)—echocardiogram showed borderline left atrial hypertrophy (LAH) and evidence of mitral stenosis (MS).

Seven years PTA—echocardiogram showed LAH, worsening MS with decreased leaflet motion.

ECG revealed atrial fibrillation.

Chest x-ray revealed LAH.

She was begun on Coumadin and a weight reduction program for chronic obesity, and a program for cigarette cessation was recommended. Surgery was considered for mitral valve replacement (MVR) but the patient was not willing, therefore, cardiac catheterization was not performed at that time.

Three years PTA—Mrs. S. began reporting episodes of breathlessness. Digoxin was added for increasing inotropy of her ventricles. Right ventricular hypertrophy (RVH) was found on echocardiogram and chest x-ray. Mrs.

S. agreed to a cardiac catheterization to evaluate valve and ventricular function.

---

### Catherization Report

Coronary arteries: insignificant, diffuse lesions
Cardiac Output: 2.5 L/minutes
Brachial Artery Pressure: 120/62 mmHg
Left Ventricular Pressure: 120/7 mmHg
Pulmonary Capillary Wedge: 27 mean pressure
Pulmonary Artery Pressure: 82/32 mmHg
Right Ventricular Pressure: 82/10 mmHg
Right Atrial Pressure: 8 mmHg
Calculated Mitral valve area: 0.6 cm$^2$
Radiocontrast material induced renal failure.

---

### Interpretation of Catherization Data

The orifice area of a normal mitral valve is about 4.5 cm$^2$. Mrs. S. shows a significant reduction down to 0.6 cm$^2$. This degree of stenosis causes a pressure gradient across the valve. The left ventricular mean pressure remains normal while left atrial and ultimately pulmonary vascular pressure rises. Her PCW is elevated, showing this change, and leads to pulmonary edema at pressures over 25 mmHg. Therefore, breathlessness arises from pulmonary hypertension with edema in its early stages.

Renal failure associated with the injection of a radiocontrast medium occasionally occurs when there is a prior history of renal insufficiency, diabetes, or impaired liver function. Mrs. S. has a long history of alcoholism.

---

6 months PTA—Mrs. S. was intubated for 3 days in acute pulmonary edema; she was put on Lasix. Pulmonary function tests after extubation showed marked reduction in airflow and volumes, both restrictive and obstructive. Atrial fibrillation persisted. Mitral valve replacement was recommended. Mrs. S. refused surgery, and was transferred to rehabilitation facility to improve general condition before returning to upstairs apartment where she lives alone. Her daughter, who lives downstairs, works all day and needs her mother to be more independent before returning home.

Table 15 lists information gleaned from a review of Mrs. S.'s current medical chart.

**Table 15. Mrs. S.'s Medical Chart Review**

| Lab values | Digoxin: | 2.0 ng/ml | | |
|---|---|---|---|---|
| | Potassium: | 4.2 mEq/L | | |
| | BUN: | 32 ng/dl | | |
| | Creatinine: | 2 mg/100 ml | | |
| | WBC: | 4,800 mm$^3$ | | |
| | RBC: | 4.0 million/mm$^3$ | | |
| | Hematocrit: | 35% | | |
| | PTT | 40 seconds | | |
| Pulmonary function test | | Observed | Predicted | Percent |
| | VC: | 3.0 L | 4.0 L | 75% |
| | FEV$_1$: | 1.8 L | 3.2 L | 59% |
| | RV: | 2.6 L | 2.0 L | 130% |
| Electrocardiogram | Atrial fibrillation; occasional PVCs; Right atrial and ventricular hypertrophy | | | |
| Chest x-ray | Left atrial, right atrial, right ventricular hypertrophy; prominent pulmonary arteries | | | |
| CAT scan | Right hemisphere, embolic event to RMCA | | | |
| Medications | Digoxin, Lasix, Coumadin, Xanax | | | |
| Echocardiogram | Mitral stenosis with mitral regurgitation; left atrial, right atrial, right ventricular hypertrophy | | | |

# FIRST PHYSICAL THERAPY VISIT

She has progressed to independent sitting tolerance and guarded transfers to wheelchair and bedside commode. She fatigues easily and routinely complains of breathlessness. Her pulse is irregularly irregular at rest and with activity.

Table 16 shows the clinical findings of the functional physical therapy evaluation.

## Interpretation of Functional Evaluation

Heart rate and rhythm were adequate for activities. Six PVCs/min is acceptable in this setting for several reasons. These include mitral valve disease and pulmonary hypertension, and right ventricular hypertension with atrial fibrillation. PVCs were previously documented in the history and did not increase in frequency or become multifocal as activity was progressed.

BP response was adaptive.

Kidney function appears to be deteriorating since her blood urea nitrogen (BUN) and creatinine values have become more elevated.

All of her respiratory symptoms indicate a severe pulmonary

Table 16. Mrs. S.'s Functional Physical Therapy Evaluation

Activities
  Rolling side to side on mat
  Supine to sit
  Sit to stand (with guarding)
  Transfer mat to chair and back (with guarding)
  Wheelchair propulsion (one arm one leg), covered 11 feet in 8 minutes with frequent rest
    periods
  Attempted ambulation in parallel bars and took 2 steps

Clinical Findings
  HR:                           90–130 bpm, atrial fibrillation and 6 unifocal PVCs per
                                  minute at rest and exercise
  BP:                           108/70 → 140/80
  RR:                           16 → 32
  RPE:                          16 at peak
  Auscultation
    Heart sounds:               S1, S2; murmurs consistent with mitral stenosis and mitral
                                  regurgitation
    Breath sounds:              Diffuse wheeze and rales
  Symptoms:                     Cough which is productive with 2 white sputum plugs
                                Fatigue and breathlessness limited ambulation

Instructions
  Mrs. S should continue bed and transfer activities.
  Endurance training program to include wheelchair propulsion in hospital hallway. This
    should be done 3-5×/day allowing rests between all functional activities. Over the next
    week, she should attempt to increase the total amount of time she works on wheelchair
    propulsion, e.g., 5 minutes, 8, 10, 12, etc., as needed, hoping to achieve 20 minute
    activity duration.
  PT will see Mrs. S. at the bedside daily to continue with therapeutic exercise for
    hemiparesis and pulmonary hygiene as needed.
  Re-evaluate for gait training in one week.

and circulatory limitation. She has chronic pulmonary hypertension which creates severe dyspnea on exertion. Her obesity presents additional load on inspiratory muscles (restrictive to lung function) and her history of smoking has damaged bronchial and alveolar structure as seen by air flow limitations and high residual volume.

The very low level of activities generating fatigue and an RPE of 16 indicate severe deconditioning and pulmonary and cardiac disease, with a reasonable motivation.

Deconditioning may be a consequence of progressive limitation of activities over some years, weakness of hemiplegia, severe cardiopulmonary disease, and renal dysfunction. Her cardiac valve, pulmonary, and renal diseases are not likely to improve. However, muscular re-education, strenghthening, and endurance training for peripheral benefits does seem possible. For these reasons, she has a low level rehabilitation prescription at this time.

Table 17. Chronology of Mrs. S.'s ICU Findings

| Measurement | Admission to ICU | 24 hours after ICU Admission |
|---|---|---|
| Vital signs | | |
| HR: | 122 | 100 |
| Rhythm: | irregularly irregular | irregularly irregular |
| BP: | 108/72 | 96/50 |
| RR: | 23 | Ventilator controlled |
| Temperature: | 102 degrees F | 100°F |
| Lab values | | |
| BUN: | Increased | Greatly increased |
| Creatinine: | Increased | Greatly increased |
| ABGs: | 66/52/7.30 ($FiO_2$ room air) | 120/54/7.32 ($FiO_2$ 100%) |
| Auscultation | | |
| Heart sounds: | Mitral stenosis/mitral regurgitation | Same |
| Breath sounds: | Diffuse wheezes and rales | Same, decreased sounds right upper quadrant |
| Chest x-ray: | Cardiomegaly, pulmonary congestion, infiltrate in RUL | Same, plus increased density of RUL; ET tube in place |
| Pulmonary capillary wedge (mmHg): | Mean 30 | Mean 42 |
| Medications: | Digoxin, coumadin, ampicillin, morphine, ranitidine | Same, plus dobutamine |

# LONG-TERM REHABILITATION AND MEDICAL EVENTS

After two more physical therapy sessions, the therapist has become aware of Mrs. S.'s increasing lethargy, fatigue, and pulmonary congestion. Her medical status has simultaneously been deteriorating. Her sputum production has increased and has become pink and frothy. Her lasix is now increased, however BUN and creatinine levels are rising as well, indicating acute renal failure. At this time, Mrs. S. is transferred to the ICU for invasive cardiopulmonary monitoring which entails insertion of a Swan-Ganz line and radial arterial line. The physician agrees that the therapist should continue to follow Mrs. S. in the ICU for assistance with pulmonary hygiene and range of motion.

Mrs. S. is intubated within 24 hours of her ICU admission for deteriorating pulmonary status, including fever and hypoxia. The therapist sees Mrs. S. twice. Treatment includes positioning, gentle vibration and endotracheal tube suctioning for greenish, thick sputum. She is too lethargic to assist with active range of motion exercises. Mrs. S. expires that night.

Table 17 lists Mrs. S.'s clinical findings while she was in the ICU.

# Interpretation of ICU Findings: What's Going on Here?

Increased lethargy, fatigue and pulmonary congestion due to two deteriorating processes: increasing renal failure as seen by BUN and creatinine values, and pulmonary edema with change in breath sounds and sputum.

Pulmonary infection developed in the ICU as seen on chest x-ray and change in sputum and breath sounds.

Suctioning, positioning, vibration done to assist secretion clearance as infection developed subsequent to pulmonary edema. Pulmonary edema alone would not be an indication for suctioning.

Drugs: Ampicillin added to fight infection. Ranitidine added to prevent GI ulcer, morphine sulfate added for pulmonary edema. Dobutamine added as an inotropic agent which assists kidney perfusion.

## SUGGESTED READING

Grossman W: Cardiac Catheterization and Angiography. 2nd Ed. Lea & Febiger, Philadelphia, 1980

# Case 5: Athletic Patient with Leg Pain, Breathlessness, Cough, Edema, Irregular Heart Beat, and Fatigue (Ms. C.)

Ms. C. is a 22-year-old female long distance runner who recently increased her training program for an upcoming competition and developed pain in both lower legs. She was evaluated by a sports medicine physician who diagnosed her with bilateral anterior compartment syndrome and referred her for physical therapy evaluation and treatment.

At the same time, she noticed wheezing and breathlessness at the end of her sprint training. She decided to discuss this breathing problem with the physical therapist.

## MEDICAL HISTORY

Ms. C.'s medical history includes frequent episodes of acute bronchitis as a child, in part attributed to her enthusiasm for outdoor winter sports. She has never smoked nor been overweight. Her blood pressure is low and her heart rate is slow and occasionally irregular. Her grandfather died of an MI at age 75 and there is no other relevant family history of heart disease.

Table 18 lists information taken from a review of Ms. C.'s medical chart.

### Interpretation of Medical Chart

1. All ECG findings are consistent with the "athlete's heart" and are due to cardiac hypertrophy, enhanced vagal tone, and decreased sympathetic drive. There is an adaptive increase in resting and exercise stroke volume allowing for a lower heart rate.
2. The chest x-ray shows similar hypertrophy due to an increase in myocardial mass.
3. Echocardiogram shows changes in cardiac dimensions that are consis-

252

**Table 18. Ms. C.'s Medical Chart Review**

| | |
|---|---|
| Physical examination | Height: 64 inches (160 cm)<br>Weight: 45 kg |
| Musculoskeletal evaluation<br>  Lower Extremities | Tenderness along tibia L > R<br>Bulging anterior compartment L > R<br>Pressure measurements:<br>  resting:  5 mmHg<br>  after 4–5 min exercise:  80 mmHg<br>  after 10 min rest:  25 mmHg |
| Vital signs | HR: 42 junctional rhythm<br>BP: 105/72<br>RR: 8 |
| Auscultation | Heart sounds: S3<br>Breath sounds: normal |
| Cough | Dry, non-productive, exercise induced |
| Lab values | ABGs: normal<br>Cholesterol: 155 mg/dl<br>  HDL: 66 mg/dl<br>  LDL: 69 mg/dl<br>  Ratio: 2.35<br>Triglyceride: 98 mg/dl<br>Hematocrit: 48%<br>Hemoglobin: 16 g/100 ml<br>Mean corpuscular volume: 98 u3 |
| Chest x-ray | Enlarged heart, increased pulmonary vascularity |
| Pulmonary function tests | VC:  110% of predicted<br>$FEV_1$:  110% of predicted<br>RV:  90% of predicted |
| 12 lead electrocardiogram | Large T wave, increased QRS complex and T wave amplitude, u wave, QT interval prolonged, QRS prolonged |
| Echocardiogram | Increased LV posterior wall thickness, increased septal thickness, increased LV chamber size |
| Medications | None |
| Social history | College student in student housing, has a steady boyfriend, is on the track team |

tent with training owing to volume loading (increased preload) of the heart, resulting in chamber enlargement and greater stretch on muscle fibers. Every contraction is more energy efficient through an enhancement of the Frank-Starling curve. Ventricular wall thickness (muscle mass) is increased due to the sustained volume overload. Thus, left ventricular end diastolic (LVED) diameter increases with a proportional increase in septal and free wall thickness to normalize wall stress.[1,2]

4. Heart Sounds. S3 is heard in aerobically-trained athletes due to the left ventricular diastolic overload.
5. Cough and breathlessness are exercise-induced, and only at high intensities. The wheezing is due to bronchospasm, induced by the stress of exercise. Her childhood history may have predisposed her to exercise-induced bronchospasm.
6. Lipids—normal and low risk for heart disease. Exercise training helps to normalize these values by increasing HDL and lowering LDL. Her fitness state may be protecting her health.
7. Blood values show athlete's adaptation to high oxygen transport capacities.
8. PFTs are resting values showing better than normal function which is consistent with her high level of training.
9. Leg pressure measurements. These are considerably elevated, consistent with anterior compartment syndrome, possibly requiring fasciotomy. Leg pressure can be measured by sphygmomanometry, using a special leg cuff big enough to encircle the calf.

## FIRST PHYSICAL THERAPY VISIT

Table 19 shows the results of Ms. C.'s initial outpatient physical therapy evaluation.

## Interpretation of Initial Outpatient Physical Therapy Evaluation

All cardiac exercise responses show a very high level of training. She was unable to reach her age predicted max HR on the bicycle (198) because she is a runner, and biking requires different pattern of LE muscle use. She experienced local muscle fatigue and exercise-induced bronchospasm on the bike test. She rated her own effort at 20 on the RPE scale.

*Metabolic responses to the first bike test.* Ms. C. was able to achieve a peak oxygen consumption ($\dot{V}O_2$) of 40 ml/kg/minute at a HR of 190, which is submaximal based on age prediction of 198. She has been training as a jogger. Consequently, she is unable to push to the same aerobic capacity as she could have done on a running test (principle of specificity of training). She is limited by bronchospasm and quadriceps fatigue. A 40 ml/kg/minute value for $\dot{V}O_2$ is excellent, especially since it is a submaximal (peak, not maximum) value. The bike test was selected with a ramp protocol in order to study her expired air gas parameters, and to control the length of the test (the lab is set up for bike, and a steady state submaximal test even on a bike with such a trained subject would be very lengthy). Most importantly, her

**Table 19. Ms. C.'s Initial Outpatient Physical Therapy Evaluation**

Activities
  Lower extremity evaluation
  Chest evaluation
  Aerobic endurance evaluation:
    Stationary bicycle exercise test, ramp protocol; no toe clips
    With and without bronchodilator, two tests, 48 hours apart

Clinical findings
  Leg evaluation
    Palpation: soft tissue bulge anteriorly and laterally, L > R; sensation in tact
    ROM and MMT: within normal limits
    History of symptom: Onset of leg pain 1½ to 2 miles at 7.5 min/mile pace; stops run after
      3–4 miles secondary to leg pain. Symptoms are consistent and reproducible with each
      run. She has noted some bulging through a defect in both anterior compartments after
      exercise and this persists until leg pain subsides and then bulging also seems to
      improve.
  Endurance evaluation

|  | Test 1 (no medication) | Test 2 (pre-medicated) |
|---|---|---|
| HR: | 42 junctional → 190 sinus tachycardia, occasional VEA | 58 sinus bradycardia → 194 sinus tachycardia, occasional VEA |
| BP: | 105/72 → 180/66 | 100/72 → 182/66 |
| RR: | 8 → 40, wheezing, breathlessness | 8 → 40, breathlessness |
| RPE: | 20 | 20 |
| RPP: | 34,200 | 35,308 |
| Workload: | 200 Watts | 225 Watts |
| Time: | 8 minutes | 9 minutes |
| METs: | 11.3 | 12.5 |
| Termination: | fatigue, wheeze, diaphoretic, breathlessness | fatigue, diaphoretic, breathlessness |
| Max $\dot{V}O_2$: | 40 ml/kg/min; 1.8 L/min | 44 ml/kg/min; 2.0 L/min |
| RQ: | 0.79 → 1.22 | 0.79 → 1.22 |
| Min Vent: | 5.2 → 45.3 L/min | 5.2 → 55 L/min |
| Tidal Vol: | 752 → 1134 ml/br | 750 → 1375 ml/br |

Chest Evaluation
  Inspection

|  | | |
|---|---|---|
| Breathing pattern: | Normal at rest, accessory muscle use at peak | Normal at rest, accessory muscle use at peak |
| Palpation | I:E 2.5 cm while wheezing; peripheral pulses forceful after exercise | I:E 5.0 cm; no wheezing; peripheral pulses forceful after exercise |

  Auscultation

|  | | |
|---|---|---|
| Heart sounds: | S3 pre- and post-exercise | S3 pre- and post-exercise |
| Breath sounds: | Inspiratory and expiratory wheeze post-exercise | Normal |
| Cough | None at rest, spasmodic and tight at peak | None at rest or with exercise |
| Medicines | Bronchodilator at end of test to reverse bronchospasm | Bronchodilator pre-test, none required after test |

Instructions
  Stop running and maintain aerobic conditioning program on stationary bicycle 5 times per
  week for 30 to 40 minutes at 85 to 90 percent max HR (× 194 bpm with bronchodilator).
  Home program: leg elevation with multiaxial ankle exercising with weights, icing before
  and after exercise, soft tissue massage before exercise.
  Visit physical therapy once a week for check on progress.

anterior compartment pain may have limited her more on a treadmill test than it did on this bike protocol.

By peak exercise, she had definitely reached her anaerobic threshold, as evidenced by her respiratory quotient value greater than 1.0, her respiratory rate, and minute ventilation. Thus muscle and metabolic fatigue are believable end points for this test. A repeat performance with bronchodilator shows marked improvement in breathing parameters and performance.

*Home Program.* On a bike program, the intensity of exercise to maintain her current high fitness level should be 85–90 percent of maximum. She may be unable to reach or maintain this intensity until her quadriceps muscles become more specifically trained for biking. The anterior compartment pain is being treated conservatively, with the hope that surgery may be avoided. She should use her bronchodilator medication prior to vigorous exercise of any type for prevention of bronchospasm and wheezing.

## POST-EVALUATION MEDICAL EVENTS

A few days after Ms. C. was first seen in physical therapy she phoned her therapist to report an increase in leg pain symptoms, the left leg pain being greater than the right leg pain. After questioning, Ms. C. admitted to attempting to run "a few miles" since she was feeling that she was deconditioning. The therapist saw her later that afternoon and detected a muscle herniation through fascia on the left leg and referred her back to her physician who found resting pressure in her left leg was now 25 mmHg and reached 80 to 100 mmHg after 1 minute of exercise. The physician determined Ms. C. should undergo left anterior compartment fasciotomy. This was done and she was referred back to physical therapy for rehabilitation.

Two weeks after surgery, she received treatments 3 times per week, consisting of ice massage for edema, ultrasound, soft tissue massage, and a strengthening and stretching program. She attempted to maintain her aerobic conditioning by using her stationary bicycle as an arm exercising device. We instructed her to pedal with her arms, 3 to 5 times per week, trying to maintain a heart rate of 85 percent of her maximum achieved heart rate of 194. She was to take her bronchodilator before aerobic exercise and was to keep her RPE between 14 to 15 for a minimum of 30 minutes. We warned her of the need to gradually progress the intensity and duration of work in order to achieve these goals.

After one month of the above program, her surgeon gave her permission to resume a brisk walking program with gradual return to jogging over the next month. She was instructed to avoid a competitive training program until three months after surgery. At that time, she would be evaluated for continued use of bronchodilators with her aerobic training program.

# Interpretation of Post-evaluation Medical Events: What's Going on Here?

Ms. C. went running against advice and developed a more acute anterior compartment syndrome as a result, which needed surgical intervention. It is possible that surgery would have been required even if she had followed a more conservative management as planned. Her zeal as a youthful, highly fit athlete led her to test her limits, which is a typical pattern for such patients.

Her orthopedic surgeon determined the severity of her anterior compartment syndrome by two methods: he took intramuscular measures of pressure both at rest and during treadmill high speed walking. Her resting and exercise intramuscular pressures were markedly elevated over normal. He also observed and could palpate the muscle herniation which occurs as the pressure rises through a slit in the fascial sheath surrounding the muscles. Exercise increases blood flow to the entire limb and causes intramuscular swelling as well as elevation in pressure. In cases such as Ms. C. represents, the fascia is too constricting for the degree of edema which develops. A slit may spontaneously appear through which muscle herniates as it swells, but recedes as it becomes quiescent. The fasciotomy releases the constriction, reduces the pressures, and totally relieves the pain. Subsequent normal function should be achieved for even the highest level of athletic requirement.[3]

Ms. C.'s condition manifested itself after she became highly trained, and then placed a higher than usual stress on her limbs with the increased intensity of training.

Physical therapy treatment for the legs was to

Decrease pain, edema, adhesions
Increase circulation, healing
Increase range of motion and strength

A conditioning program for her arms was set to a very high intensity because Ms. C. was starting at such a high initial value of training. Her arms were certainly not previously trained, so that there was little expectation that she would be able to meet the prescription for intensity until she had "trained" the local arm muscles to do this form of work. This implies that her cardiopulmonary fitness level would detrain to some degree inevitably, and could only fully retrain when she resumed running at her former speed, duration, and frequency. With detraining, her heart size would decline, her resting heart rate would rise, her ventricular muscle wall thickness would decrease, and her S3 would probably disappear. Her ECG "abnormalities" would disappear and she would show a much normalized ECG even as her heart "regressed".

Ms. C. has exercise-induced asthma. This is a condition which will not likely improve no matter how hard she trains. Bronchodilator therapy is a symptomatic approach to treatment, but it works very effectively to permit exercise and training to proceed. If she decides not to progress her training to the higher level, she can do very well, as shown by her exercise capacity on her test performed without the bronchodilator.

## REFERENCES

1. Huston T P, Puffer J C, Rodney W M: The Athletic Heart Syndrome, N Engl J Med 313:24, 1985
2. Wenger N, Gilbert C: The athlete's heart. In Hurst JW (ed): The Heart, Arteries, and Veins. 3rd ed. McGraw-Hill, New York, 1974
3. Mubarak S J, Hargens A R: Compartment Syndromes and Volkmann's Contracture. Saunders' Monographs in Clinical Orthopedics. Vol. 3. W B Saunders, Philadelphia, 1981

# Glossary

| | |
|---|---|
| ABG | Arterial blood gas |
| ADL | Activities of daily living |
| aVF | Augmented limb lead of ECG—foot |
| B/K | Below knee |
| BP | Blood pressure |
| BPM | Beats per minute |
| BUN | Blood urea nitrogen |
| CABG | Coronary artery bypass graft |
| CAD | Coronary artery disease |
| CCU | Coronary care unit |
| CHF | Congestive heart failure |
| COPD | Chronic obstructive pulmonary disease |
| CPK | Creatine phosphokinase |
| CVA | Cerebrovascular accident |
| ECG | Electrocardiogram |
| ECHO | Echocardiography |
| EF | Ejection fraction |
| ER | Emergency room |
| ETT | Exercise tolerance test |
| $FEV_1$ | Forced expiratory volume in one second |
| GBPS | Gated blood pool study |
| HDL | High-density lipoproteins |
| HR | Heart rate |
| IABP | Intra-aortic balloon pump |
| ICU | Intensive care unit |
| LAD | Left anterior descending (coronary artery) |
| LAH | Left atrial hypertrophy |
| LCx | Left circumflex (coronary artery) |
| LE | Lower extremity |
| LDH | Lactate dehydrogenase (lactic [acid] dehydrogenase) |
| LDL | Low-density lipoproteins |
| LV | Left ventricle |
| LVED (P or V) | Left ventricular end diastolic (pressure or volume) |
| LVEF | Left ventricle ejection fraction |
| MI | Myocardial infarction |

| | |
|---|---|
| MMT | Manual muscle test |
| MS | Mitral stenosis |
| $M\dot{V}O_2$ | Myocardial $O_2$ consumption |
| MVR | Mitral valve replacement |
| PAC | Premature atrial contraction |
| PCW | Pulmonary capillary wedge |
| PFT | Pulmonary function test |
| PND | Paroxysmal nocturnal dyspnea |
| PTA | Prior to admission |
| PTCA | Percutaneous transluminal coronary angioplasty |
| PTT | Prothrombin time |
| PVC | Premature ventricular contraction |
| PVD | Peripheral vascular disease |
| $\dot{Q}$ | Cardiac output |
| RBC | Red blood cell |
| RCA | Right coronary artery |
| RLE | Right lower extremity |
| RMCA | Right middle cerebral artery |
| ROM | Range of motion |
| RPM | Revolutions per minute |
| RPE | Rating of perceived exertion |
| RPP | Rate-pressure product |
| RR | Respiratory rate |
| RUL | Right upper lobe |
| RV | Right ventricle |
| RVH | Right ventricular hypertrophy |
| SDU | Step down unit |
| SGOT | Serum glutamic-oxaloacetic transaminase |
| SL | Sublingual |
| SPM | Steps per minute |
| ST | S–T segment on ECG |
| TNG | Trinitroglycerol (nitroglycerin, coronary vasodilater) |
| UBE | Upper body exerciser (Cybex) |
| VC | Vital capacity |
| $V_D/V_T$ | Dead space to tidal volume ratio |
| VEA | Ventricular ectopic activity |
| $\dot{V}_E$ | Minute ventilation |
| $\dot{V}O_2$ | Oxygen consumption |
| WBC | White blood cell |

# APPENDIX

**Table A-1. Normal Laboratory Values**

| Determination | Normal Values | |
|---|---|---|
| | **Male** | **Female** |
| Complete blood count | | |
| Hematocrit (Hct) | 42–52% | 37–48% |
| Hemoglobin (Hbg) | 13–18 g/100 ml | 12–16 g/100 ml |
| Erythrocyte (RBC) | 4.2–5.9 million/mm$^3$ | |
| Mean corpuscular volume (MCV) | 86–98 u$^3$ | |
| Mean corpuscular hemoglobin (MCH) | 28–33 μg | |
| Mean corpuscular concentration (MCC) | 32–36% | |
| Total eosinophil count | 70–440/mm$^3$ | |
| Leukocyte (WBC) | 4,300–10,800 mm$^3$ | |
| Differential count | | |
| Polys | 40–75% | |
| Bands | 0–4% | |
| Lymphocytes | 20–45% | |
| Monocytes | 2–10% | |
| Eosinophils | 1–6% | |
| Basophils | <1% | |
| Reticulocyte count | 0.5–2.5% | |
| Erythrocyte sedimentation rate (ESR) | 1–3 mm/hr | 1–20 mm/hr |
| Platelet count (PLT) | 150,000–350,000/mm$^3$ | |
| Prothrombin time (PT) | within 2 seconds of control | |
| Partial thromboplastin time (PTT) | 25–40 seconds | |
| Thrombin time (TT) | within 5 seconds of control | |
| Bleeding time test | 2–9.5 minutes | |
| Fibrin split products | 1:4 or less | |
| Glucose (fasting) | 65–110 mg/dl | |
| Hemoglobin A1C | 3.8–6.4% (non–diabetic range) | |

*(Continued)*

Table A-1. (*Continued*)

| Determination | Normal Values | |
|---|---|---|
| | Male | Female |
| Cholesterol | 120–220 mg/dl | |
| Triglyceride | 40–150 mg/dl | |
| High density lipoproteins (HDL) | 30–65 mg/dl | 35–80 mg/dl |
| Low density lipoproteins (LDL) | 70–190 mg/dl | |
| Very low density lipoproteins (VLDL) | <40 mg/dl | |
| Total cholesterol/HDL | <4.0 | |
| Creatinine phosphokinase (CPK) | 17–148 U/ml | 10–79 U/ml |
|    MB band | <5% | |
| Lactate dehydrogenase (LDH) | 45–90 U/ml | |
| Serum glutamic–oxaloacetic transaminase (SGOT) | 7–27 U/ml | |
| Potassium (K+) | 3.5–5.2 mEq/L | |
| Sodium (Na+) | 136–145 mEq/L | |
| BUN | 8–25 mg/dl | |
| Creatinine | 0.7–1.5 mg/100 ml | |
| Calcium | 8.5–10.5 mg/dl | |
| Iron | 50–150 μg/dl | |
| Uric acid | 3.0–7.0 mg/dl | |
| Lactic acid | 0.6–1.8 mEq/L | |
| Oxygen saturation | 94–100% | |
| $PaO_2$ | 80–100 mmHg | |
| $PaCO_2$ | 35–45 mmHg | |
| pH | 7.35–7.45 | |
| Digitalis | | |
|    Digoxin | 0.5–2.5 ng/ml | |
|    Digitoxin | 20–35 ng/ml | |
| Quinidine sulfate | 5–8 mg/l | |
| Procainamide | 4–8 mg/l | |
| Lidocaine | 1–6 mg/ml | |
| Protein bound iodine | 4–8 μg/dl | |
| Serum thyroxine ($T_4$) | | |
|    total | 4–11.5 μg/dl | |
|    free | 0.8–2.4 ng/dl | |
| Serum $T_3$ concentration | 80–100 ng/dl | |
| Serum thyroid stimulating hormone | 5–10 μU/ml | |

# Index

Page numbers followed by t represent tables; those followed by f represent figures.